T0297654

Xerostomia

An Interdisciplinary Approach to Managing Dry Mouth

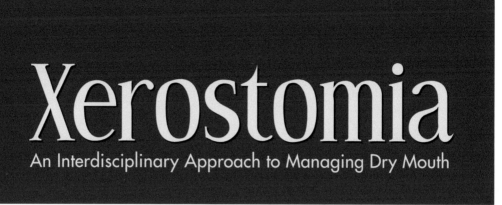

Xerostomia
An Interdisciplinary Approach to Managing Dry Mouth

Edited by

Sarah M. Ginsberg, EdD, CCC-SLP, F-ASHA
Department of Special Education and
Communication Sciences and Disorders
Eastern Michigan University
Ypsilanti, Michigan

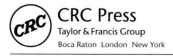

CRC Press
Taylor & Francis Group
Boca Raton London New York

CRC Press is an imprint of the
Taylor & Francis Group, an **informa** business

Xerostomia: An Interdisciplinary Approach to Managing Dry Mouth includes ancillary materials. Included are patient web resource pages. Please visit www.routledge.com/9781630914899 to obtain access.

Cover Artist: Lori Shields

First published 2020 by SLACK Incorporated

Published 2024 by CRC Press
2385 NW Executive Center Drive, Suite 320, Boca Raton FL 33431

and by CRC Press
4 Park Square, Milton Park, Abingdon, Oxon, OX14 4RN

CRC Press is an imprint of Taylor & Francis Group, LLC

Library of Congress Cataloging-in-Publication Data

Names: Ginsberg, Sarah M., 1966- editor.
Title: Xerostomia : an interdisciplinary approach to managing dry mouth /
[edited by] Sarah M. Ginsberg.
Description: Thorofare, NJ : SLACK Incorporated, [2020] | Includes
bibliographical references and index.
Identifiers: LCCN 2020003661 (print)
ISBN: 9781630914899 (paperback)
Subjects: MESH: Xerostomia
Classification: LCC RC815 (print) | NLM WI 230 | DDC
616.3/1--dc23
LC record available at https://lccn.loc.gov/2020003661

ISBN:9781630914899(pbk)
ISBN: 9781003526995(ebk)

DOI: 10.1201/9781003526995

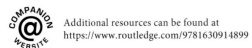

Additional resources can be found at
https://www.routledge.com/9781630914899

DEDICATION

In profound appreciation for my exemplars of patient-centered care:
Arthur W. Tai, MD;
Theron L. Dobson, MD;
Kevin M. Sloan, DDS, MS;
and my father, David J. Ginsberg, MD

CONTENTS

Acknowledgments

This text was first and foremost a work by great clinicians, many of whom are also great researchers and educators. These professionals enjoy the benefit of having their names associated with their hard work through the inclusion of their names on their chapters. However, there were a number of people without whom this book would have been less than it is, and their names do not appear on any chapters.

My deepest gratitude to:

- Patricia J. Sallans, BS, graduate speech-language pathology student, for your participation, insights, and collegiality in conducting the study
- Olivia M. Martin, BS, graduate speech-language pathology student, for your support in all things writing and web resource related
- Daniel S. Kopas, BBA, for your graphic design guidance on the patient resource pages
- Cathy M. DeRuiter, MA, CCC-SLP, colleague and extraordinary reader, for your eagle eye and insights

And most importantly:

- Jeffrey K. More, my patient husband. No one who is not a clinician should ever have to listen to as much information about xerostomia as you did.

ABOUT THE EDITOR

Sarah M. Ginsberg, EdD, CCC-SLP, F-ASHA is a Professor of Communication Sciences and Disorders at Eastern Michigan University in Ypsilanti, Michigan. She teaches dysphagia, her primary area of clinical interest, as well as clinical and diagnostic methods in speech-language pathology. She has published extensively in the area of the scholarship of teaching and learning. She is the coauthor of *Scholarship of Teaching and Learning in Speech-Language Pathology and Audiology: Evidence-Based Education* and is the founding editor of *Teaching and Learning in Communication Sciences & Disorders.*

Contributing Authors

Rebecca H. Affoo, PhD, CCC-SLP, SLP(C), Reg. CASLPO (Chapters 3 and 6)
Assistant Professor
School of Communication Sciences and Disorders
Faculty of Health
Dalhousie University
Halifax, Nova Scotia, Canada

Michael A. Blasco, MD (Chapter 4)
Fellow
Department of Otolaryngology–Head and Neck Surgery
Princess Margaret Cancer Centre/University Health Network
University of Toronto
Toronto, Ontario, Canada

Yusuf Dundar, MD (Chapter 3)
Department of Otolaryngology–Head and Neck Surgery
Wayne State University
Detroit, Michigan

Lea E. Erickson, DDS, MSPH (Chapter 5)
Professor
Associate Dean for Education and Student Life
School of Dentistry
University of Utah
Salt Lake City, Utah

Jeffrey M. Hotaling, MD (Chapters 3 and 4)
Assistant Professor
Department of Otolaryngology–Head and Neck Surgery
Wayne State University
Detroit, Michigan

Sharon Ingersoll, PharmD (Chapters 3 and 8)
School of Nursing
Nebraska Methodist College
Omaha, Nebraska

Joseph Murray, PhD, CCC-SLP, BCS-S (Chapters 3 and 6)
Audiology and Speech Pathology Service
VA Ann Arbor Healthcare System
Ann Arbor, Michigan

Kristine Tanner, PhD, CCC-SLP (Chapter 7)
Associate Professor
Department of Communication Disorders
Brigham Young University
Provo, Utah

Bryan Trump, DDS, MS (Chapter 5)
Associate Professor
Board Certified Oral and Maxillofacial Pathologist
School of Dentistry
University of Utah
Salt Lake City, Utah

INTRODUCTION

Brief Xerostomia Overview

At the risk of oversimplifying at the beginning of this text for the purposes of a brief overview, *xerostomia* is defined as a condition in which there is a sensation that there is not enough saliva to keep the mouth moist (Locker, 2003; National Institutes of Health, 2014). One of the conundrums of this condition is that, although it can be objectively measured in patients who have a decrease in the flow of their saliva, thus indicating true salivary gland hypofunction, not all patients who report concerns regarding a dry mouth will have an objectively measured decrease in their flow rate and as such, have complaints of xerostomia in the absence of hypofunction. We see that although patients with a significant decrease in measures of their saliva are more likely to complain of dry mouth, it is not a one-to-one correlation of flow rate and patient perception. Patients with normal production of saliva may also complain of oral dryness, potentially indicating difficulties with the quality of the saliva. Thus, we need to concern ourselves with the subjective as well as the objective in treating patients who have concerns about dry mouth. Both concerns are addressed in this text.

Xerostomia has many possible causes, including diabetes, Parkinson's disease, Sjögren's syndrome, cancer treatments, HIV/AIDS, and nervous system damage. Additionally, there are countless medications that can cause xerostomia. Many patients experience xerostomia due to taking a large number of medications that can cause dry mouth as a side effect. Xerostomia affects one in four individuals, with the incidence increasing in people over the age of 50 (Ramirez-Sepulveda et al., 2016). The data suggest that millions of people around the world likely suffer from xerostomia due to the wide range of associated medical conditions and medications (Strietzel et al., 2006).

Xerostomia can cause an array of disorders, including increased tooth decay, oral infection, and difficulty communicating, chewing, and swallowing (American Dental Association, 2015). Research suggests that patients with severe dry mouth are at risk for voice disorders, particularly throat clearing, dry throat, difficulty with voice projection, and discomfort with vocal use (Liu, Masterson, Srouji, Musonda, & Scott, 2012; Tanner et al., 2015). They are also at risk for significant declines in their quality of their life as a result of the xerostomia (Locker, 2003; Slade & Spencer, 1994).

Overcoming Challenges of Managing Xerostomia

In the world of science and medicine, the research regarding xerostomia is relatively new. The first large-scale studies were published in the 1980s, and the momentum has continued to increase as our understanding of the needs for the assessment and management of patients with xerostomia continues to improve (Sreebny & Vissink, 2010). However, from both the research and clinical practice, we continue to see that providing effective care for patients with xerostomia is far from simple and straightforward. There are numerous challenges that are faced in caring for individuals with xerostomia. These include a lack of research in a number of disciplines that address patient complaints, the continued perspective by nondental professionals that oral health is solely the domain of dental professionals, and the mistaken perspective that xerostomia is a relatively negligible problem that does not impact patients' quality of life.

This text addresses the evaluation and management of patients with xerostomia in detail from the perspective of specialists in each area for the purpose of informing colleagues within and across the disciplines of all health care providers (HCPs) about the complex impact of xerostomia on individuals' health, quality of life, and ability to function. The intent is for this information to be consumed by a wide range of HCPs. In order to be effective in caring for our patients, we need to have a clear understanding of how the condition impacts them.

The patient perspective is included in this text as well because this is a critical, and often over-looked, perspective. We all benefit from understanding the patient experience. There are many individuals with xerostomia who are feeling adrift and dissatisfied with their care. Their frustrations at finding well-informed, interested, and caring HCPs were the primary motivation behind creating this text. Although the chapters are written for professionals, most chapters have corresponding patient web resources that can be found at www.routledge.com/9781630914899 The patient-friendly materials include resources for patients that will provide them with information to help them understand more about their condition and will facilitate working as partners with their HCPs. These resources are available to all disciplines for the purposes of better informing ourselves and our patients. By understanding the full impact of xerostomia and the role that professionals can play in supporting patients and each other, we can improve their outcomes. The best care that we can provide for our patients with xerostomia is compassionate, interdisciplinary, and patient centered.

References

Liu, Z. W., Masterson, L. M., Srouji, I. A., Musonda, P., & Scott, D. G. (2012). Voice symptoms in patients with autoimmune disease: A cross-sectional epidemiological study. *Otolaryngology–Head and Neck Surgery, 147*(6), 1108-1113.

Locker, D. (2003). Dental status, xerostomia, and the oral health-related quality of life of an elderly institutionalized population. *Special Care in Dentistry, 23*(3), 86-93.

National Institutes of Health. (2014). Dry mouth (xerostomia). National Institute of Dental and Craniofacial Research. Retrieved from https://www.nidcr.nih.gov/oralhealth/topics/drymouth

Ramirez-Sepulveda, K., Murillo-Pedrozo, A., Zuluaga-Villegas, D., Vasco-Grajales, K., Posada-Lopez, A., & Agudelo-Suarez, A. A. (2016). Perceptions of patients with xerostomia about quality of life, general and oral health: A qualitative study. *Global Journal of Health Science, 8*(11), 257-269. doi:10.5539/gjhs.v8n11p257

Slade, G. D., & Spencer, A. J. (1994). Development and evaluation of the oral health impact profile. *Community Dental Health, 11*(1), 3-11.

Sreebny, L. M., & Vissink, A. (2010). *Dry mouth, the malevolent symptom: A clinical guide.* Ames, IA: Wiley-Blackwell.

Strietzel, F. P., Martin-Granizo, R., Fedele, S., Lo Russo, L., Mignogna, M., Reichart, P. A., & Wolff, A. (2007). Electrostimulating device in the management of xerostomia. *Oral Diseases, 13*(2), 206-213. doi:10.1111/j.1601-0825.2006.01268.x

Tanner, K., Pierce, J. L., Merrill, R. M., Miller, K. L., Kendall, K. A., & Roy, N. (2015). The quality of life burden associated with voice disorders in Sjögren's syndrome. *Annals of Otology, Rhinology, and Laryngology, 124,* 721-727.

Xerostomia Patient Pages

Patient web resource pages can be found at www.routledge.com/9781630914899 They will provide patients with information to help them understand more about their condition, and will facilitate working as partners with health care providers. These resources are available to all disciplines for the purposes of better informing ourselves and our patients.

- Introduction to Xerostomia: Xerostomia definition, symptoms, causes, and related professionals
- Advocating for Yourself as a Patient: Being prepared for your appointment to get the most out of it
- Choosing a Doctor: Finding a health care provider who will be a good fit
- Questions Are the Answer: Questions to consider for before, during, and after your appointment
- Otolaryngologists Explain Xerostomia: Understand anatomy, possible evaluations, and treatment
- Dental Care and Dry Mouth: Strategies for dental care and reducing discomfort
- Dry Mouth and Eating: Impact of dry mouth on eating and tips for improvements
- Hydration Protocol for Voice: Tips to keep your throat and vocal cords hydrated
- Working With Your Pharmacist: Medication information and management strategies

INTERDISCIPLINARY PATIENT-CENTERED CARE FOR PATIENTS WITH XEROSTOMIA

Sarah M. Ginsberg, EdD, CCC-SLP, F-ASHA

In order to provide the best care for our patients with xerostomia, we need to provide them with interdisciplinary, patient-centered care (PCC). The key to effective interdisciplinary care is accepting that all health care providers (HCPs) bear some degree of responsibility for examining the oral cavity and not assuming it is a dentist's job alone. PCC includes providing care that "explores patients' reasons for visiting the physician, understanding medical issues, and emotional needs, increasing prevention and health initiatives, and enhancing the relationship between patients and providers" (Wanzer, Booth-Butterfield, & Gruber, 2004, p. 364).

INTERDISCIPLINARY ORAL HEALTH CARE

Since the early 2000s, there has been a movement toward the interdisciplinary or interprofessional delivery of health care in order to facilitate communication and effective patient care (Bridges, Davidson, Odegard, Maki, & Tomkowiak, 2011). The purpose of teams of HCPs working together is to improve patient outcomes. With the Patient Protection and Affordable Care Act, movement began within the United States to incentivize improved quality of care delivered as efficiently and economically as possible (Boynes, Lauer, Deutchman, & Martin, 2017; Nester, 2016). The intention of providing the best patient outcomes at the lowest cost is most likely achieved through the use of interdisciplinary teamwork. In order to be effective, teams of HCPs, including physicians, dentists, speech-language pathologists, and pharmacists, working together must demonstrate the ability to work together for the "purposes of coordinating care and education for their patients; improving overall patient health; promoting self-care; identifying and treating health conditions sooner rather than later; and helping patients effectively manage chronic health conditions" (Nester, 2016, p. 128).

The successful function of teams of HCPs from a range of different disciplines requires autonomy, communication, and respect across members. In 2000, the U.S. Surgeon General produced a report on oral health in the United States calling on HCPs to recognize that the mouth provides us with a "window" on an individual's general health status, noting that "as the gateway of the body,

Ginsberg, S. M. (Ed.).
Xerostomia: An Interdisciplinary Approach to Managing Dry Mouth (pp. 1-8).
© 2020 Taylor & Francis Group.

the mouth senses and responds to the external world and at the same time reflects what is happening deep inside the body" (U.S. Department of Health and Human Services, 2000, p. 10). Not only can the mouth be considered the window to the body's overall health, but also it is known that oral health is integral to good general health (Yellowitz, 2016).

Unfortunately, oral care continues to be siloed in many health care contexts and is considered the sole domain of dentists by many HCPs, including physicians (Folke, Fridlund, & Paulsson, 2008). It has been reported that physicians and nurses largely skip examining the oral cavity during the examination of the head and neck, which otherwise includes an assessment of the eyes, ears, nose, and throat (Haber et al., 2015; Yellowitz, 2016). The process of providing quality care regarding the mouth is further eroded by poor communication between medical and dental professionals. This may be due to a variety of factors, including the lack of representation of dental providers in health care teams, inadequate numbers of dental professionals, and limited bidirectional communication between medicine and dentistry (Boynes et al., 2017). As a result, medical HCPs seldom collaborate with oral health professionals (Yellowitz, 2016). Poor communication between medicine and dentistry combined with limited or nonexistent oral health assessments by nondental HCPs may pose a barrier to the optimal delivery of patient care for individuals with xerostomia. Limited assessment and communication between these groups of HCPs can contribute to errors in the delivery of proper medication and inaccuracies of medication records, delayed findings of disease that could aid in diagnosing systemic conditions, and low prioritization of oral health problems.

There are a significant number of systemic diseases, which are more specifically addressed in later chapters of this text, that include important oral symptoms, including xerostomia. As noted previously, oral health is known to be an indicator of overall general health. Poor oral health is associated with many conditions that, when left untreated, can result in decreased general health (Yellowitz, 2016). Creating an interdisciplinary oral health workforce would increase the focus and prioritization of oral health and oral care. The inclusion of oral health evaluations by an entire team of HCPs across disciplines would facilitate timely patient access to better coordinated care, resulting in improved patient outcomes.

PATIENT-CENTERED CARE

Health care has seen a dramatic paradigm shift in the relationship between HCPs and patients. Before the late 1970s and 1980s, there was little discussion regarding the relationship between the two groups, and the balance of power was clearly in the hands of the educated, knowledgeable physician, nurse, dentist, or speech-language pathologist. However, as late as 1977, a disagreement is documented in the literature between psychiatrists and the rest of medicine regarding whether the consideration of patients beyond the realm of their testable and treatable biology was relevant to medical care (Engel, 1977). Engel argued that with the accepted medical model of that time, medicine was in "crisis" as a result of the view that disease was only defined in terms of "somatic parameters" and that "physicians need not be concerned with psychosocial issues" (p. 129). The alternative proposed, the biopsychosocial model, which took into account the patient, his or her social environment, and access to support resources including health care, started to take hold in medicine and gained momentum in the 1980s.

By 1988, the Picker/Commonwealth Program for Patient-Centered Care adopted the phrase *patient-centered care* as a way to call attention to the need for HCPs to shift their focus away from the purely biological nature of disease and incorporate attending to the patients' and their family's needs (Barry & Edgman-Levitan, 2012). By the early 2000s, the Institute of Medicine (IOM) established the importance of PCC in maintaining a quality of patient care in the United States (Barry & Edgman-Levitan, 2012; Epstein & Street, 2011; IOM, Committee on Quality of Health Care in America, 2001). At the core of PCC lies the notion that although HCPs are the experts in the science and art of implementing their discipline's tools and knowledge, patients are the experts regarding

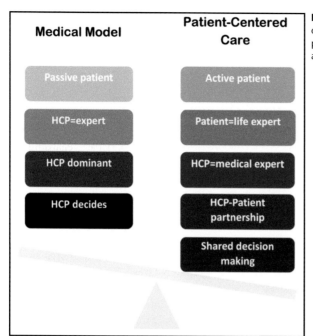

Figure 1-1. The medical model vs. PCC. Elements of the medical model contrast with PCC because patients and HCPs work toward determining approaches to assessment and treatment.

their own experiences, cultures, values, and preferences. Thus, the delivery of care to the patient (and the family) must be "respectful of and responsive to individual patient preferences, needs, and values, and ensuring that patient values guide all clinical decisions" (IOM, Committee on Quality of Health Care in America, 2001, p. 3). This represents a dramatic shift away from the paternalistic medical model in which patients were the passive recipients of health care and moved them toward partners in their own care. Engel (1977) noted that this means that the patient gets to decide if his or her condition represents an "illness" or "problems of living" (p. 133). In essence, the PCC model shifts the expectations and balance for participation and communication between HCPs and patients (Figure 1-1).

The PCC model implies that HCPs will hold respect for their patients' views and decisions regarding their care. It also suggests that there will be open dialogue, effective communication, and sensitivity in the partnership between HCPs and patients. The goal of that partnership should include shared decision making, empathy, and collaboration (Epstein & Street, 2011). Because patients have the ability and the right to make decisions once leaving the HCPs' office related to taking medications, modifying behaviors, or accepting any recommendations, health care can never be effective without patient engagement (Greenfield, Kaplan, Ware, Yano, & Frank, 1988). In chronic illness, it is inevitable that patients will self-manage their condition as they make decisions about their health-related activities on a daily basis (Bodenheimer, Lorig, Holman, & Grumbach, 2002). Even in the face of generally good health, we all make decisions from day to day regarding exercise or flossing our teeth due to fatigue, distraction, or a multitude of different reasons in which we may ignore our HCPs' advice about optimum behaviors. Therefore, it is in our best interest when working with those who are not generally healthy to come to recommendations for assessment and care that the patient feels are beneficial and appropriate to his or her scenario in order to maximize the likelihood of participation and best/better outcomes.

Care that effectively incorporates patient participation and input has been demonstrated to be more effective in decreasing the functional limitations of patients relative to their condition and disease activity and improving their health-related quality of life compared with care that relies on the medical model (Brown et al., 2002; Greenfield et al., 1988). Furthermore, increasing a patient's sense of control and autonomy regarding his or her decision making is likely to result in better outcomes.

PCC has not only been shown to improve patient outcome measures, but also it has been correlated with improved patient satisfaction and is likely to decrease the patient's stress associated with the disease (Brown et al., 2002; Epstein & Street, 2011).

Challenges

There are two significant challenges to the implementation of PCC: patients and HCPs. This may appear self-evident; however, the data suggest that the effectiveness of the patient–provider relationship and collaboration is dependent on specific characteristics of each. It is not safe to assume that all patients are interested in playing an active role in their health care. Research suggests that patients who are younger are more likely to be active participants in their care than older patients, women are more likely to take an active role than men, and patients with higher education are more likely to be actively engaged in their care process than those without college educations (Arora & McHorney, 2000). Patients with chronic illness may be more engaged in daily self-management and collaborative decision making than those with acute or severe illness (Arora & McHorney, 2000; Bodenheimer et al., 2002; Brown et al., 2002). It is also worth noting that some patients merely prefer to take a passive role in their health care (Brown et al., 2002; Epstein & Street, 2011; Greenfield et al., 1988). The reasons for this may include personality, communication style, anxiety regarding health outcomes, and cultural differences. Although a preference or expectation for passivity exists in some patients, the data from the literature would suggest that the next generation of patients, beginning with baby boomers and continuing through younger patients, are less and less likely to take passive roles in their health care. On a more forward note, data suggest that many of the individuals presenting with xerostomia are middle-aged women (i.e., more active participants in their health care), particularly secondary to autoimmune diseases. Many of these women have access to internet-based resources and want and expect to have an active role in their xerostomia-related care.

The second half of the equation for an effective and collaborative relationship in health care is the HCPs. Given that the medical model continues to be pervasive in many educational and clinical settings, it should be no surprise that there are HCPs who are resistant to a PCC approach to care, which requires them to be less dominant. It may be that the role of collaborator instead of controller is uncomfortable or unfamiliar. Several studies have demonstrated that when patients attempt to engage in active discussion regarding decision making, physicians can demonstrate irritation, frustration, and anxiety and engage in a "battle of wills" in order to regain control of the interaction (Brown et al., 2002; Greenfield et al., 1988). The willingness of highly educated and experienced professionals in health care to accept that they are not in the position of holding all of the knowledge needed to make an effective decision for the patient can represent a considerable shift in self-perception and how they view their role. However, for the sake of improved patient outcomes, it is critical that HCPs learn to relinquish the sense of unquestioned authority that they may have been taught and begin to see themselves as partners in care.

Shared Decision Making

As partners in care under the PCC model, we need to invite our patients to engage in collaborative or shared decision making. The concept of shared decision making embodies for some the pinnacle of PCC and represents an exchange of information from both parties (Barry & Edgman-Levitan, 2012, p. 780). In working toward a shared decision, the clinician provides the patient with recommendations or options alongside the relative advantages and disadvantages of each choice for managing his or her condition. The patient must in turn share values and preferences that he or she is weighing in considering each option to come to an acceptable and feasible solution. Although many of our patients with xerostomia have limited options regarding their treatment, engaging them in this model of deliberate discussion and fostering a sense of shared decision making will help them to understand specifically what their options are and help them feel more actively engaged in their own care.

For patients who come to HCPs with a view of themselves as actively engaged patients with a strong sense of their own desire to be a partner in their own care, it may not be necessary to encourage the patient toward shared decision making. However, for patients who are uncertain about what their role is in the decision-making process or for those who prefer to remain passive, it is the responsibility of the HCPs to provide them with education about their role and the value of their participation in the discussion (Barry & Edgman-Levitan, 2012; Bodenheimer et al., 2002; Elwyn et al., 2012; Towle & Godolphin, 1999). We must provide that encouragement to facilitate patients expressing themselves and asking questions. If we do not hear patients' voices, we do not understand what their goals are, how well they understand their condition or the options that we have laid out for managing it, or what is feasible for them to undertake in the way of management. Without hearing their perspective, we are likely to make invalid assumptions regarding how their condition impacts the quality of their lives and their priorities. If we fail to understand what is important and vital to our patients, we are likely to make recommendations for assessment or treatment that will be ignored. By creating opportunities for our patients to openly share with us that they are not willing to undertake an assessment or participate in a given treatment approach, we increase the chances that our patients will have positive health and quality of life outcomes.

For example, I can recommend to my patient with dysphagia that he stop drinking liquids altogether to avoid pneumonia due to his chronic aspiration. If, in providing this recommendation, I do not foster an opportunity for him to tell me that he is unwilling to take this measure to avoid aspiration, then I send him away unarmed with any knowledge about alternatives. Furthermore, if I find out that he develops aspiration pneumonia once back at home due to drinking liquids, I might be tempted to label him as "noncompliant" and irrational because he did not follow my directions. The concept of compliance returns us to the medical model in which the clinician holds all of the knowledge and power and presumes a judgment of failure or personal flaw on the part of the person who does not follow through with his or her directions (Barry & Edgman-Levitan, 2012: Bodenheimer et al., 2002; Towle & Godolphin, 1999). On the other hand, if I use a PCC approach with my patient, I can present him with options for treatment that lay out for him the level of relative risk of aspiration compared with the relative quality of life that can be retained based on his stated values. If we have a relationship of mutual respect and understanding, I can support his decision-making process. With appropriate education and information provided to him, he may make a decision for maintaining a moderately reasonable quality of life and continue drinking fluids under a protocol that he can live with at the expense of incurring greater risk of aspiration and yet maintain appropriate hydration for skin integrity and other bodily function needs. After providing him with information, I would check for his understanding of the ramifications of his choices and document both the discussion and his preferences. Although his choice might not be, in my mind as a clinician, the best choice for keeping his lungs free of infection, I want to know what he is going to choose at home and counsel him on the second-best option rather than send him away ignorant of his views and his intention to disregard recommendations. In this PCC-based approach, I have listened to him as a partner in the care process and respected his expertise regarding his own life. The concept of judging my patient as noncompliant no longer fits with my view and understanding of him and his choices.

Given the critical role of shared decision making in PCC, as well as the resistance some HCPs have shown, it is worth considering how we can facilitate shared decision making with our patients. One way that we can support our patients in shared decision making is to provide them with education and knowledge regarding their condition and their choices (Bodenheimer et al., 2002; Elwyn et al., 2012; Towle & Godolphin, 1999). Educational materials may come in the form of written materials, support groups, professionals in other disciplines, videos, or online resources, such as those associated with this text (www.routledge.com/9781630914899). The use of instructive materials with patients can result in increased knowledge, decisions that are more consistent with the patients' values, better understanding of risks, and decreased passivity of patients (Barry & Edgman-Levitan, 2012). When we attempt to educate patients, we also need to check on their understanding as well as their cognitive and emotional reactions to what they have learned (Brown et al., 2002). As patients develop a greater understanding of their disease and their options for managing it, they are more likely to feel confident engaging in discussions about it with their HCPs.

The second way that we can support our patients in engaging in shared decision making is to foster the discussions that will move the process forward with input from both participants. We may need to explicitly encourage input and invite dialogue. It may be unfamiliar to the patient to have HCPs who demonstrate caring about his or her opinion. In order to engage in shared decision making, there are eight specific competencies or steps that HCPs should consider as an overview of the process (Towle & Godolphin, 1999):

1. Establish a partnership foundation with the patient.
2. Identify the patient's preferred levels and forms of information.
3. Learn what role the patient sees him- or herself taking in his or her own care as well as who else he or she might want involved in decision making.
4. Listen to the patient's concerns regarding the condition and expectations he or she has about management.
5. Identify choices that are available to the patient, considering what fits with what you have learned about him or her and what he or she has expressed.
6. Help the patient understand the options available, helping him or her weigh advantages and disadvantages of each relative to the knowledge you have gained about him or her.
7. Navigate the negotiation of what his or her preferences are balanced with your recommendations through the partnership you have formed.
8. Come to an agreement on the final plan and begin implementation.

In Chapter 2, we discuss specific strategies for improving the quality of communication in PCC care, thus improving patients' satisfaction with their care. Here we briefly discuss a framework for PCC clinical practice that applies specifically to shared decision making. Elwyn et al. (2012) described the deliberation model for moving the dialogue with patients forward. In this model (Figure 1-2), HCPs are encouraged to support the deliberation process through three steps: choice talk, option talk, and decision talk. In choice talk, HCPs make sure that patients are aware of the choices that they have available to them. In this step, education and discussion, noted previously, are critical to helping patients understand the options and what they represent. The second step of option talk moves patients toward a greater depth of understanding about their options, including checking for their understanding, considering risks and benefits, and double-checking through teach back in which patients are given the opportunity to explain and teach the clinician what they have learned and how they conceptualize their options (Elwyn et al., 2012, p. 1364). Finally, decision talk focuses on the choices that patients make and confirms that they are ready and comfortable with the final decision. Working to be sure that patients understand what their options are, no matter how limited, and that we, as HCPs, will support their deliberation process through our partnership with them will not only increase their satisfaction with their care, but also it will continue to foster a positive and productive relationship with us as they continue to have their many health care needs addressed.

New models of patient care mean shifting the relationship between the HCP and the patient from one that was unidirectional and dominated by the professional (i.e., the provider is the expert who informs the patient that this is what will be done) to one that is more bidirectional. The PCC model acknowledges that each person in the relationship, including those representing each discipline, brings expertise to the table. HCPs come with technical knowledge, experience, and specific skills, whereas patients bring their insights, values, and preferences into what it is like to live with a condition and how they cope with it from day to day (Clark et al., 2008). The adoption of this model improves the quality of care able to be delivered as well as the outcomes our patients are likely to experience. As we collectively grapple with the assessment and management of a condition such as xerostomia, which often has no cure, we can improve patients' experiences as they navigate the complexities of their health issues. We can also increase their satisfaction with the care that they receive

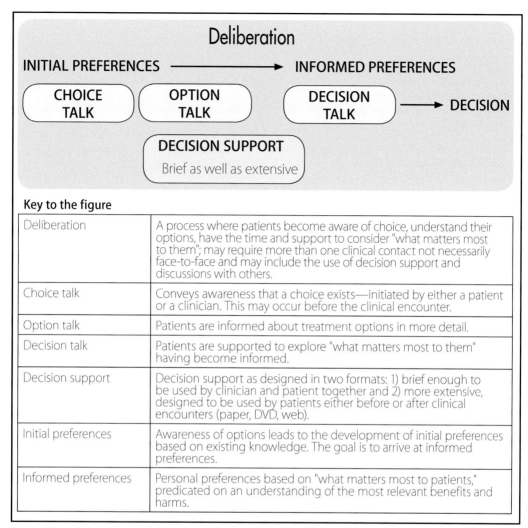

Figure 1-2. A shared decision-making model. The use of a stepwise deliberation process between HCPs and patients in order to facilitate shared decision making effectively. (Reprinted with permission via Attribution 2.0 Generic [CC BY 2.0] from Elwyn, G., Frosch, D., Thomson, R., Joseph-Williams, N., Lloyd, A., Kinnersley, P., … Barry, M. [2012]. Shared decision making: A model of clinical practice. *Journal of General Internal Medicine, 27*[10], 1361-1367. doi:10.1007/s11606-012-2077-6)

and with the quality of their lives as they manage their conditions. Future chapters detail some of the barriers and suggest problem-solving solutions and tools to help move toward successful partnering and long-term rewards for patients with xerostomia and other health-related issues.

REFERENCES

Arora, N., & McHorney, C. (2000). Patient preference for medical decision making: Who really wants to participate? *Medical Care, 38*(3), 335-341.

Barry, M. J., & Edgman-Levitan, S. (2012). Shared decision making—The pinnacle of patient-centered care. *New England Journal of Medicine, 366*(9), 780-781.

Bodenheimer, T., Lorig, K., Holman, H., & Grumbach, K. (2002). Patient self-management of chronic disease in primary care. *Journal of the American Medical Association, 288*(19), 2469-2475.

Boynes, S. G., Lauer, A., Deutchman, M., & Martin, A. B. (2017). An assessment of participant-described interprofessional oral health referral systems across rurality. *Journal of Rural Health, 33*(4). 427-437. doi:10.1111/jrh.12274

Bridges, D. R., Davidson, R. A., Odegard, P. S., Maki, I. V., & Tomkowiak, J. (2011). Interprofessional collaboration: Three best practice models of interprofessional education. *Medical Education Online, 16.* doi:10.3402/meo.v16i0.6035

Brown, R., Butow, P., Henman, M., Dunn, S., Boyle, F., & Tattersall, M. (2002). Responding to the active and passive patient: Flexibility is the key. *Health Expectations, 5*(1), 236-245.

Clark, N., Cabana, M., Nan, B., Gong, M., Slish, K., Birk, N., & Kaciroti, N. (2008). The clinician-patient partnership paradigm: Outcomes associated with physician communication behavior. *Clinical Pediatrics, 47*(1), 49-57.

Elwyn, G., Frosch, D., Thomson, R., Joseph-Williams, N., Lloyd, A., Kinnersley, P., … Barry, M. (2012). Shared decision making: A model of clinical practice. *Journal of General Internal Medicine, 27*(10), 1361-1367. doi:10.1007/s11606-012-2077-6

Engel, G. (1977). The need for a new medical model: A challenge for biomedicine. *Science, 196*(4286), 129-136.

Epstein, R. M., & Street, R. L. (2011). The values and value of patient-centered care. *Annals of Family Medicine, 9*(2), 100-103. doi:10.1370/afm.1239

Folke, S., Fridlund, B., & Paulsson, G. (2008). Views of xerostomia among health care professionals: A qualitative study. *Journal of Clinical Nursing, 18*(6), 791-798. doi:10.1111/j.1365-2702.2008.02455.x

Greenfield, S., Kaplan, S., Ware, J., Yano, E., & Frank, H. (1988). Patient's participation in medical care: Effects on blood sugar control and quality of life in diabetes. *Journal of General Internal Medicine, 3*(5), 448-457.

Haber, J., Hartnett, E., Allen, K., Hallas, D., Dorsen, C., Lange-Kessler, J., … Wholihan, D. (2015). Putting the mouth back in the head: HEENT to HEENOT. *American Journal of Public Health, 105*(3), 437-441.

Institute of Medicine, Committee on Quality of Health Care in America. (2001). *Crossing the chasm: A New health system for the 21st century report brief.* National Academies Press. Retrieved from https://pubmed.ncbi.nlm.nih.gov/25057539

Nester, J. (2016). The importance of interprofessional practice and education in the era of accountable care. *North Carolina Medical Journal, 77*(2), 128-132. doi:10.18043/ncm.77.2.128

Towle, A., & Godolphin, W. (1999). Framework for teaching and learning informed decision making. *British Medical Journal, 319*(7212), 766-769. doi:10.1136/bmj.319.7212.719

U.S. Department of Health and Human Services. (2000). *Oral health in America: A report of the Surgeon General.* Rockville, MD: U.S. Department of Health & Human Services, National Institute of Dental and Craniofacial Research, National Institutes of Health.

Wanzer, M., Booth-Butterfield, M., & Gruber, K. (2004). Perceptions of health care providers' communication: relationships between patient-centered communication and satisfaction. *Health Communications, 16*(3), 363-384. doi:10.1207/ S15327027HC1603_6

Yellowitz, J. A. (2016). Building the ideal interdisciplinary team to address oral health. *Journal of the American Society on Aging, 40*(6), 60-65.

2

LIVING WITH XEROSTOMIA

Sarah M. Ginsberg, EdD, CCC-SLP, F-ASHA

As we consider the variety of signs and symptoms that patients with xerostomia may present with, we need to consider the impact of the condition on their quality of life and give credence to their concerns. Increasing our understanding of how health care providers (HCPs) view patients with xerostomia, xerostomia management, and what patients with xerostomia are looking for from us will help us be more effective in providing them with effective care.

SIGNS AND SYMPTOMS

Xerostomia can be objectively confirmed by determining if there is true salivary gland hypofunction with a significant decrease in the flow rate (Frydrych, 2016; Villa, Connell, & Abati, 2015; Zunt, 2018). However, xerostomia is defined as a "subjective complaint of dry mouth" (Villa et al., 2015, p. 45), suggesting that it is not always associated with an objectively measurable decrease in salivary flow and making patient concerns a critical component in the diagnosis and management of xerostomia (Frydrych, 2016; Villa et al., 2015). It has been noted that patients who experience a decrease in the flow rate over 50% are more likely to experience signs and symptoms of dry mouth than those with a less than 50% decreased flow rate (Napenas, Brennan, & Fox, 2009; Zunt, 2018).

The patient experience of xerostomia is likely to be highly individualized and does not always correlate directly with salivary flow. The concerns that patients express extend greatly beyond what may be thought of as a simple dry mouth requiring extra hydration. Patient worries may include dental problems, challenges with eating, disrupted sleep, communication difficulties, and psychosocial concerns. Many of the signs and symptoms represent daily challenges for patients with xerostomia and are summarized in Table 2-1.

These signs and symptoms could represent a decrease in the oral health of patients. Good oral health "enables the individual to speak and socialize without active disease, discomfort, or embarrassment which contributes to general well-being" (Kay & Locker, 1997, p. 8). The impact of dry mouth on individuals' daily lives can be quite substantial. The effects of xerostomia have been

Ginsberg, S. M. (Ed.).
*Xerostomia: An Interdisciplinary Approach
to Managing Dry Mouth* (pp. 9-27).
© 2020 Taylor & Francis Group.

Table 2-1. Signs and Symptoms of Xerostomia

AREA	SIGN	SYMPTOM	SOURCES
Oral cavity	• Halitosis • Poor denture and prosthesis retention • Ulceration from dentures • Mucositis • Gingivitis • Dental caries and erosion • Loss of dentition • Cheilitis • Lingual surface changes • Increased frequency of infection • Dry appearance • Mucosa susceptible to trauma • Instruments stick to mucosa	• Stomatodynia (burning mouth syndrome) • Chronic dryness requiring liquids and stimulants • Denture discomfort	• Frydrych, 2016 • Guggenheimer & Moore, 2003 • Napenas et al., 2009 • Villa et al., 2015 • Zunt, 2018
Swallowing/deglutition	• Compromised nutrition • Dysphagia • Weight loss • Pneumonia	• Dryness when eating • Difficulty swallowing • Alternate liquids and solids when eating • Taste disturbances • Acidic and spicy food intolerance • Avoidance of dry or crunchy foods	• Guggenheimer & Moore, 2003 • Napenas et al., 2009 • Rogus-Pulia & Logemann, 2011 • Villa et al., 2015 • Zunt, 2018
Voice/communication	• Dysphonia (hoarseness)	• Throat clearing • Difficulty projecting voice • Vocal discomfort • Throat soreness • Avoidance of singing	• Folke, Paulsson, Fridlund, & Soderfeldt, 2009 • Tanner et al., 2015 • Zunt, 2018 *(continued)*

Table 2-1 (continued). Signs and Symptoms of Xerostomia

AREA	SIGN	SYMPTOM	SOURCES
Sleep		• Dryness when waking • Disrupted sleep	• Folke et al., 2009 • Ngo, Thomson, Nolan, & Ferguson, 2016 • Rydholm & Strang, 2002
Psychosocial	• Avoidance of socialization • Avoidance of shared meals	• Decreased pleasure with socializing • Embarrassment • Decreased self-esteem and confidence • Anxiety • Demoralization syndrome	• Folke et al., 2009 • Ngo et al., 2016 • Rydholm & Strang, 2002

referred to as an "aggravating misery" based on the "devastating and debilitating" signs and symptoms (Folke et al., 2009, p. 245) and a "significant burden" for patients (Villa et al., 2015, p. 45) and can cause significant challenges to perceptions of well-being. Qualitative studies, ideally suited to understanding patients' personal experiences from their perspective (Denzin & Lincoln, 2003), have suggested that the level of frustration posed by the condition can be overwhelming. Because xerostomia has a strong potential to impact the individual's sense of psychological and physical well-being, it is critical that all HCPs are able to appreciate some of the hardships patients living with xerostomia endure on a daily basis.

Isolation is a consideration that may affect the daily life of individuals with xerostomia. Persons experiencing communication frustration secondary to xerostomia may exhibit decreased willingness to socialize. Interpersonal communication may feel disrupted due to difficulties articulating clearly and the frequent need to sip, which can disrupt the flow of communication (Folke et al., 2009; Ngo et al., 2002). The inability to project their voice, particularly in loud or group communication settings, may also contribute to a sense of discomfort with socialization. Individuals with xerostomia describe the inability to sing, which for some deters them from participation in a preferred leisure activity, such as singing in church choirs. As a result of the feelings of isolation, illness, and changes in functioning, patients may experience demoralization syndrome due to a strong sense of helplessness and the inability to control symptoms (Rydholm & Strang, 2002).

Eating difficulties and discomfort with shared meals may further contribute to patient loneliness. The need to constantly sip water throughout a meal, slow chewing, oral pain, and food avoidance may all create discomfort and anxiety for patients with xerostomia when eating in a group or in public settings (Owens, Gibson, Periyakaruppiah, Baker, & Robinson, 2014; Rydholm & Strang, 2002). Problems with eating secondary to xerostomia can result in compromised nutrition, weight loss, and swallowing, further compromising quality of life (Guggenheimer & Moore, 2003; Napenas et al., 2009; Villa et al., 2015; Zunt, 2018).

Poor quality of sleep due to xerostomia was noted to be a critical factor in the decision to stop working, which may diminish quality of life, particularly in individuals who are not mentally prepared to separate from their vocation or are dependent on their income (Folke et al., 2009; Owens et al., 2014; Rydholm & Strang, 2002). Patients who experience such a disrupted pattern of sleep may feel chronically fatigued. This fatigue coupled with underlying and contributing xerostomia-like disease factors, such as Sjögren's syndrome, depression, and cancer treatments, can lead to exhaustion that may impede individuals from feeling that they can continue to be effective in their jobs. Unfortunately, poor sleep quality influences how well a person is able to think and communicate and thus becomes a cyclical problem. Therefore, the challenges of communication may impact individuals' work lives and also cause them to discontinue employment. Ceasing employment has the potential to heighten their sense of isolation.

ORAL HEALTH-RELATED QUALITY OF LIFE

Given the varied aspects of daily life that can be debilitating for patients with xerostomia and the potential for it to compromise their sense of well-being, researchers set out to measure the impact of xerostomia on patients' quality of life. One way to accomplish this was to look at a model of health-related quality of life (HRQOL) controls that examines factors beyond the objective disease process. HRQOL considers aspects of a patient's ability to function with a condition and takes into account the economic, social, and emotional impact of the condition (Ferrans, Zerwic, Wilbur, & Larson, 2005; Wilson & Cleary, 1995). An example of the characteristics an HRQOL model can consider include the individual's biological condition, symptoms, support systems, personality, and the environment in which he or she resides or functions.

There are a wide variety of HRQOL models available in the literature. The original models proposed have been adapted and updated over time. With the advent of the World Health Organization's development of the *International Classification of Functioning, Disability and Health* (ICF; World Health Organization, 2002), a model of HRQOL can be adapted. Because "quality of life is influenced by the extent we feel capable of participating in activities that meet our needs and expectations," the view of HRQOL through the ICF model seems particularly appropriate (Folke et al., 2009, p. 246). In Figure 2-1, we can consider this new integrated model that acknowledges the components of both the early oral health–related quality of life (OHRQOL) models and the ICF model as it applies to xerostomia. The advantage of such a model is that it moves away from a medical model in which the person is viewed solely as a person in a disease or disability state and moves us toward the biopsychosocial model, which allows HCPs to have a more comprehensive view of the patient (World Health Organization, 2002). Furthermore, the ICF model components give us a mechanism to identify how, for our patients with xerostomia, the condition may be viewed as a disability and have a negative influence on their sense of self (Owens et al., 2014). Considering the OHRQOL variables can facilitate our assessment and management of all aspects of the individual.

In this model, the original conceptualization of an OHRQOL view is honored by beginning with the biological function of the individual because this typically is the foundational factor that leads patients and their team of HCPs toward decisions that may ultimately improve the quality of the patients' lives. Although disease states are often objective and measurable, the patients' experiences and perceptions of life with the disease are not, but they still need to be considered. Thus, their experiences with symptoms, such as the struggle to soothe oral discomfort or to project their voice, will be influenced by their individual characteristics, such as how they view themselves and how much they understand about their disease. Factors in the environment, including the ability to access social support and dietary limitations, can also impact how they experience and respond to symptoms. Individual characteristics will also influence patients' decision making about their functioning level, including what activities they believe they are able to complete and participating in life events, such as sharing meals with friends and speaking in public. The inclusion of patients' general

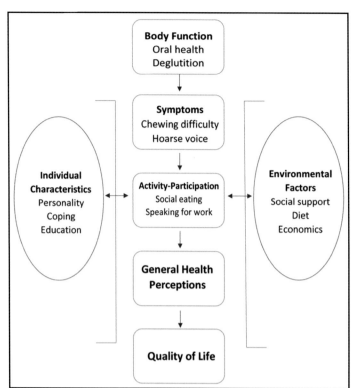

Figure 2-1. A model of OHRQOL: an integrated model of HRQOL (Adapted from Ferrans, C., Zerwic, J., Wilbur, J., & Larson, J. [2005]. Conceptual model of health-related quality of life. *Journal of Nursing Scholarship, 37*[4], 336-347; Wilson, I., & Cleary, P. [1995]. Linking clinical variables with health-related quality of life. *Journal of the American Medical Association, 273*[1], 59-65; and World Health Organization. [2002]. *Towards a common language for functioning, disability and health.* Retrieved from https://www.who.int/classifications/icf/icfbeginnersguide.pdf?ua=1)

health perceptions as a consideration is based on the understanding that how patients perceive their overall general health is a strong indicator of the use of health-related services as well as a predictor of mortality (Ferrans et al., 2005; Wilson & Cleary, 1995). Although it is typically the HCPs' primary concern to focus on biological function in evaluating and treating diseases, it will be most beneficial to a patient if the more holistic view of the patient and his or her related factors are considered.

The relevancy of an OHRQOL model's applicability to oral health has been extensively researched. In considering oral diseases such as xerostomia, we can conceptualize that the symptoms and negative experiences associated with the xerostomia may compromise overall mental and physical functioning in a manner that could lessen the patients' quality of life (Locker, 2003). Several patient questionnaire tools have been created to assess OHRQOL issues. One such mechanism that can help HCPs to focus particularly on oral issues and their potential impact on the quality of life of patients with xerostomia is the use of the Oral Health Impact Profile (OHIP; Slade & Spencer, 1994). Developed in the early 1990s, the OHIP was the first attempt at measuring the impact of OHRQOL. The OHIP, as noted by the authors of the measure, could be valuable for (a) allowing practitioners to focus on the most immediate needs of patients when combined with clinical data; (b) improving the consideration of patients' oral health–related behaviors, including engaging in preventative and treatment-related aspects of care; and (c) fostering insights into oral health that allows us to advocate for dental and oral health aspects of care to be integrated into the domain of patient health outcomes rather than seeing them as separate and unrelated factors.

Although the original OHIP questionnaire was demonstrated to be valid and reliable, it is lengthy, at 49 items. Questions focus on the domains of patients' perceptions of functional limitations, pain, psychological discomfort, physical disability, psychological disability, social disability, and their quality of life. Questions in the OHIP-14 regarding patients' perceptions of a handicap (e.g., life generally less satisfying or unable to function) may parallel the OHRQOL item of general health perception (see Figure 2-1). The OHIP-14 is a shorter version of the original OHIP with only two questions from each domain included from the original lengthier version (Table 2-2). It has been used widely in studies of patients with xerostomia after being validated and published (Slade, 1997). Using the OHIP-14, patients in Norway with xerostomia secondary to a primary diagnosis of Sjögren's syndrome were found to have increased oral distress and associated decreased HRQOL (Enger, Palm, Garen, Sandvik, & Jensen, 2011). In New Zealand, strong positive responses on all items of the OHIP-14 were found to be positively associated with younger adult patients with xerostomia (Thomson, Lawrence, Broadbent, & Poulton, 2006). Older Japanese patients were identified as having increased scores (indicating lower quality of life) on the OHIP-14 in association with xerostomia (Ikebe et al., 2007).

The research using the OHIP-14 questionnaire demonstrates that patients across regions and ages experience a decrease in their OHRQOL in the presence of xerostomia. Although the OHIP-14 has been particularly well established as a reliable and valid tool and used in research, it is not the only instrument available and potentially useful for HCPs. Additional sets of questions regarding patients' perceptions of oral dryness and its impact on functioning have been implemented in research and found to be not only statistically significant but also useful in aiding HCPs in understanding the presence and impact of xerostomia in patients (Villa et al., 2015).

HEALTH CARE PROVIDERS' VIEWS OF XEROSTOMIA MANAGEMENT

Despite the literature demonstrating the pervasive impact that xerostomia can have on patients' quality of life, HCPs appear uncertain as to how to address and manage the condition independent of the etiology. Folke, Fridlund, and Paulsson (2008) interviewed HCPs, including physicians, dentists, and nurses, regarding their understanding and management of xerostomia. Findings suggested that providers were aware of the potential negative impact of xerostomia on patients' quality of life due to dental decay, chronic discomfort, and eating and swallowing difficulties, as well as the possible negative impact of xerostomia on social interactions, including communication and sharing of meals. HCPs were found to have an indifferent attitude toward the problem despite some awareness of the far-reaching impact xerostomia may have on their patients. The providers in the study considered xerostomia to be a trivial problem that did not warrant sufficient attention because xerostomia may be considered a subjective difficulty and not in their scope of practice. HCPs were either not empathetic to the problems or were inadequately prepared to manage the condition and, as a result, were likely to avoid discussing it with patients or colleagues. Xerostomia was not consistently evaluated by HCPs and was not considered critical. Furthermore, it was assumed that other professionals would address it, which justified their lack of knowledge about the clinical management of xerostomia on the assumption that it was not their responsibility.

Research has been conducted to investigate the knowledge, attitudes, and practices of a variety of HCPs in relation to xerostomia care. Perhaps not surprisingly, there is some variability across disciplines and contexts regarding how HCPs approach patients with xerostomia. However, there is consistency in the finding that all professionals indicate that they do not have enough formal education and knowledge about xerostomia to feel confident about their skills.

Studies of physicians' views of xerostomia suggest that they have a fair awareness of the condition and its potential to have a severe impact on a patient's oral health and that oral health can have an impact on a person's general health and quality of life (Andersson, Furhoff, Nordenram, & Wardh, 2007; Appleby, Temple-Smith, Stacey, Bailey, & Deveny, 2016; Folke et al., 2008). General

Table 2-2. Oral Health Impact Profile

IN THE LAST SIX MONTHS	NEVER	HARDLY EVER	OCCASIONALLY	FAIRLY OFTEN	VERY OFTEN
1. Have you had trouble pronouncing any words because of problems with your teeth, mouth, or dentures?					
2. Have you felt that your sense of taste has worsened because of problems with your teeth, mouth, or dentures?					
3. Have you had painful aching in your mouth?					
4. Have you found it uncomfortable to eat any foods because of problems with your teeth, mouth, or dentures?					
5. Have you been worried by dental problems?					
6. Have you felt tense because of problems with your teeth, mouth, or dentures?					
7. Has your diet been unsatisfactory because of problems with your teeth, mouth, or dentures?					
8. Have you had to interrupt meals because of problems with your teeth, mouth, or dentures?					
9. Have you found it difficult to relax because of problems with your teeth, mouth, or dentures?					
10. Have you been a bit embarrassed because of problems with your teeth, mouth, or dentures?					
11. Have you been a bit irritable with other people because of problems with your teeth, mouth, or dentures?					
12. Have you had difficulty doing your usual jobs because of problems with your teeth, mouth, or dentures?					
13. Have you felt that life in general was less satisfying because of problems with your teeth, mouth, or dentures?					
14. Have you been totally unable to function because of problems with your teeth, mouth, or dentures?					

Reprinted with permission from Slade, G. D. (1997). Derivation and validation of a short-form oral health impact profile. *Community Dental Oral Epidemiology, 25,* 284-290.

practice physicians in these studies demonstrated an understanding that xerostomia may be seen more frequently in patients with autoimmune diseases and older adults, particularly related to polypharmacy. Physicians held opinions ranging from the notion that dry mouth is a trivial problem that "individuals have to endure and cope with" (Folke et al., 2008, p. 794) to the idea that it is a significant problem but one that was "not my department" (Andersson et al., 2007, p. 126). One physician summarized that because dry mouth is subjective and it may be based on the patient's perception, "it is impossible for a health care provider to objectively measure such a feeling," believing that it is the "patient's state of mind" (Folke et al., 2008, p. 794). Few physicians were systematic about assessing the oral cavity, and most typically conducted the examination only when the patient complained of pain in the head or throat. Reasons cited for not assessing the oral cavity, in addition to it not being their department, included that they did not have enough time, it was a low priority condition, or they were inadequately educated about the problem. Most physicians in these studies indicated that they did not attempt to manage patients' xerostomia but might refer the patient to a dentist, although many reported that they did not. Not all physicians indicated that they would consider a change in medication due to complaints of dry mouth. Occasional management recommendations given by physicians included the use of saliva substitutes and drinking more water. Some physicians reported giving general advice to their patients that could in fact be harmful to oral health, such as the use of hard candy without specifying that it should be sugar free or the use of high citric acid items, such as "sucking on lemons," which can be corrosive to dentition (Appleby et al., 2016, p. 904).

Comparable with physicians, nurses participating in studies of oral health knowledge with older adults demonstrated inadequate knowledge and limited ability to manage issues of oral care (Ek, Browall, Eriksson, & Eriksson, 2018; Preston, Punekar, & Gosney, 2000). The majority of nursing and nursing assistants acknowledged that oral care was important, but in cases in which patients were in residential scenarios or were not independent in self-care, there was a lack of systematic methods of ensuring the completion of oral care. Nursing staff cited time constraints as one of the reasons that oral care was not completed. Participating nurses also reported that they had a lack of knowledge regarding oral health and thus were not confident regarding managing oral issues. The nurses' knowledge about oral health and oral care was not always correct (Preston et al., 2000). When they did give suggestions to patients, it was most commonly related to denture care.

Although professionals from medicine and nursing may consider xerostomia to be the dentists' area of concern, dentists may not be in agreement. General practice dentists did not always attend to xerostomia and symptoms presented by patients (Folke et al., 2008; Sreebny & Valdini, 1988). Some dental health professionals consider the matter of dry mouth to be insignificant and inconsequential. A study of dentists in Scotland found that not all participants had correct knowledge regarding xerostomia nor did they all feel that it was important to treat it (Abdelghany, Nolan, & Freeman, 2011). To date, there is no literature available indicating that speech-language pathologists are actively engaged in the assessment and management of xerostomia specifically. The inspection and observation of xerostomia are primarily noted during an oral mechanism evaluation that is completed for the purposes of assessment of speech, voice, or swallowing.

PATIENT SATISFACTION WITH HEALTH CARE PROVIDERS

Patients' Perceptions

Given the complex experience of the patient with xerostomia and the lack of apparent knowledge and ownership of HCPs working with patients suffering from this condition, it would appear that there is a high potential for dissatisfaction with the quality of health care for these patients. There are very few studies that have included patients' perspectives on their health care as part of their research. In the existing studies, patients have identified frustrations with their HCPs as contributing to a negative overall experience of living with xerostomia. Patients in Sweden experienced little to no empathy from their HCPs regarding their frustration with xerostomia (Folke et al., 2009). In fact, patients reported an awareness that their HCPs considered them to be "whining and annoying" and were dismissive when they attempted to have their xerostomia addressed (Folke et al., 2009, p. 250). In Colombia, individuals with Sjögren's syndrome experienced inattention to their xerostomia symptoms from their caregivers and were often given little educational information regarding their condition, leaving them discontented with their care (Ramirez-Sepalveda et al., 2016). The authors noted that limitations in the national health care system likely contributed to patients' frustration.

Investigation Into Patient Satisfaction With Health Care Providers

As there have been so few investigations into patients' satisfaction with HCPs, with virtually none conducted in the United States, a new study was conducted for the purpose of inclusion in this text. This study was conducted by this chapter author to specifically investigate the satisfaction of individuals with xerostomia regarding their care.

Methods

A qualitative study was conducted with 15 participants in the United States who self-identified as having xerostomia. Participants were recruited through xerostomia-specific social media outlets and through professional referrals from HCPs. Thirteen participants had been diagnosed with Sjögren's syndrome, and two of the participants experienced xerostomia secondary to medications. The average age of the 14 women and 1 man participating in the study was 64 years old. All lived independently in their own homes, and none were dependent on care providers.

In accordance with the approved institutional review board methods, each participant was audio recorded during an individual interview that was semistructured and used open-ended questions. Key questions asked participants what types of health care professionals they had consulted in managing their xerostomia and how satisfied they had been with their care. They were also asked what they would like HCPs to know about caring for patients with xerostomia. Data were analyzed at the sentence level in the context of the individual's narrative to identify initial codes. Because codes were analyzed for patterns and themes, they were "linked together" to begin identifying emerging themes from the overlap of related codes that are supported by the verbatim narratives found within individual transcripts labeled with pseudonyms (Denzin & Lincoln, 2003, p. 279).

Results

Participants voiced frustration with their experiences with members of their health care team. Although there were a few who shared positive experiences from interactions with HCPs, most of the interactions were sources of aggravation, with one participant saying, "It makes me so mad; if I could spit, I would!" Three main sources of dissatisfaction were voiced by participants: (a) dismissive responses, (b) delegitimizing responses, and (c) limited empathy and listening. Finally, participants want their HCPs to "just listen" to them and be patient centered.

Dismissive Responses

Comments from HCPs who were dismissive of patients' concerns included suggesting to Beth that "your symptoms are just a nuisance." Rebecca raised concerns about managing her xerostomia during a hospitalization but found that her concerns were "dismissed." Esther shared that when she was finally diagnosed, her physician said, "Yes, you have Sjögren's syndrome," and then he "patted me on my head and sent me away" with no information. She noted that "you go to the doctor and you tell them stuff, some doctors will poo-poo you." Hannah felt that her dentist was more concerned about the cavities and root canals, and "they consider dry mouth a minor issue." Lucinda shared that when she tried to discuss her symptoms with her dentist, "he just wouldn't listen to me."

Kathleen sought out an otolaryngologist for support for her xerostomia. "He sat there with his arms crossed and he said, 'there is nothing we can do to help you.' Then he looked at my tongue and said, 'looks normal to me.'" Jenny Lee said that she had been told by a number of HCPs "'It's just dry mouth and that's no big deal; a lot of people have dry mouth.' They don't see the bigger problems that you have." Judith, an academic in a health-related field, recounted her frustration with a dentist who would not discuss a treatment strategy with her:

> I found some literature about new advances in treatment for oral decay, but I also found information from Sjögren's programs, like Johns Hopkins Sjögren's Center, that had the recommendations that they gave their patients for oral care. I shared all of it with her. She did not acknowledge any of the information that I sent her, but she was thrilled to tell me that she had found xylitol mints for me. I asked her if that was the sum of her plan to get ahead of my oral decay problems. She offered that she supposed I could come in more frequently to have my teeth cleaned too. I found a new dentist.

Delegitimizing Responses

A number of the participants suggested that worse than being dismissive of their symptoms, some HCPs actually suggested that the problems were the patients' fault or that it was just in their head. A number of participants shared that although their HCPs did not actually come out and say it, they felt they were being judged as being "nuts." Kathleen noted that when she tried to discuss her xerostomia, she had the feeling that her HCP thought she was "a hypochondriac. They don't say it but … but we don't get any further along in the conversation, let me put it that way." Caroline related that as she was trying to talk with a new physician about her dry mouth, "he said 'well, why don't we have a psychiatrist talk to you about these problems?' I just said 'goodbye.'" Beth went to see her physician for swelling in her salivary glands prior to being diagnosed with Sjögren's syndrome. "He asked me if I was making this up which, at the time, I thought … well, why would anyone make this up? It's not like you can make up swollen salivary glands; they are huge." Lucinda shared that when she repeatedly presented with "rampant caries" to her previous dentist, he "accused me of not taking care of my teeth properly."

Limited Empathy and Listening

Dissatisfaction was experienced by participants who felt that they were not listened to or cared about. Dianne reflected that her physician was willing to offer a prescription drug for her xerostomia, but she noted that she could not engage him further in discussion, observing "I'm not sure he is that interested." Lucinda shared of a dentist she had seen that "wouldn't listen when I would complain about irritations or something." Esther related that none of her HCPs have ever asked what she has done to manage her xerostomia symptoms, stating that her participation in this study was her first experience being asked about it. Caroline shared a perspective with a number of participants who felt that "a lot of dentists are not receptive to anything other than what they were told when they went to dental school." Interestingly, Caroline was a person who had done enough of her own research to understand the components of saliva, but she could not convince her dentist to listen to her.

"Could You Just Listen?"

When asked what they would like from their HCPs, Caroline's comments were representative of most of the participants when she said "Could you just listen and not give a flip who you are? Could you just listen and say 'What you said is important and let's see if we can deal with these issues'?" When she did find an HCP who would listen to her, she noted her satisfaction that "whenever I say 'I have this problem' … he listens to me talk about it," and he tries to find resources for her. Esther added she would like to ask HCPs to "please ask me about it. Please talk to me and listen to me when I say 'this worked for me.'" Lucinda wanted all HCPs to treat her the way her new dentist does because he says to her "Tell me, explain it to me," and he listens to her when she talks about living with xerostomia. Beth shared that she found a "great dentist" who "has learned everything she can

… and [is] finding out from her other [xerostomia] patients what works for them." Rebecca wanted HCPs to "be more open to what is being said by the patient as opposed to what they think they know. It would be more patient-centered instead of self-centered."

The results of this study are consistent with previous research. The dismissive and delegitimizing attitudes described are similar in nature to the HCPs' trivializing, indifferent, not-my-problem, and it-is-in-their-head views of xerostomia described as cited earlier in this chapter (Andersson et al., 2007; Folke et al., 2008, 2009; Sreebny & Valdini,1988). In the process of recruiting participants with xerostomia for this study, a colleague suggested that "… none of them are satisfied," implying that patient dissatisfaction is a reflection of the lack of a cure for many. However, data from studies of patient satisfaction with HCPs suggest that dissatisfaction is not clearly related to a lack of a definitive cure.

Interspersed with stories of dissatisfaction with HCPs, there were stories of professionals who did indeed make the individual feel listened to and cared about. Patients who perceived that they had accessible and empathetic HCPs were more likely to hold a favorable view of their health care than those who did not find their providers to be empathetic to their condition. There was significant value to them in "'being understood' through listening" (Ngo et al., 2016, p. 6). Results from this study confirm that participants were more likely to be satisfied when they felt that someone listened and cared.

This begs the question of why so many HCPs are disregarding or invalidating their patients' concerns and not listening to them empathetically. It may be that xerostomia is being "neglected" due to time constraints, low prioritization of the problem, and not being the patient's primary concern (Folke et al., 2008, p. 796). It might also be that perceiving that xerostomia management is not within their scope of care and practice causes the HCPs to either not listen or not ask about the condition. Previous studies suggested that there was general awareness of OHRQOL (Andersson et al., 2007; Appleby et al., 2016; Folke et al., 2008); however, it is unknown how widespread HCPs' awareness of the quality of life impact factor is for xerostomia in the United States. Although we cannot be certain as to why xerostomia matters are being dismissed, whether as unimportant or not worthy of the visit time, a lack of knowledge about xerostomia could be a viable explanation as to why a professional would attempt to delegitimize patient concerns as being fabricated or "in their head." The research described within this chapter gives plausible explanations as to why HCPs respond as they do to concerns regarding xerostomia. However, we can work to ensure that all HCPs are armed with the tools and knowledge that will improve their patients' outcomes and satisfaction with care. The data from the participants in all of the studies to date indicate that patients are not asking to be cured of an often-incurable condition in order to be more satisfied, but they are looking to their HCPs for a different type of response from the one many have received.

How Do We Improve Patient Care and Satisfaction?

Better Education of All Health Care Providers

In order to address the disconnect between general health care and oral care, the Institute of Medicine recommended that disciplines outside of the dental profession develop competencies in the ability to screen oral health (Dolce, 2014). There is a need to develop an "interprofessional oral health workforce" (Haber et al., 2015, p. 437) such that oral mechanism examinations are routinely conducted as part of the head and neck examinations completed by HCPs (Boynes et al., 2017; Dolce, 2014; Yellowitz, 2016). Core competencies have been suggested in this literature for nondental professionals to be able to conduct oral cancer screenings and recognize the presence of dental caries, periodontal disease, and xerostomia. Professionals who have been educated in the ability to screen oral health would also be in a position to counsel patients regarding oral care and make referrals to dental professionals.

In order to improve the quality of care for patients with xerostomia, we need to begin to address the underlying deficit that appears to exist in the education of most HCPs. To date, the research has been reasonably conclusive that a change in how we educate HCPs would improve the care of patients with xerostomia. Studies suggest the need for improved education of physicians (Andersson et al., 2007; Appleby et al., 2016; Folke et al., 2008). Research from the nursing literature also suggests that patients' oral health care suffers partially because of a lack of knowledge on the part of the nurses (Ek et al., 2018; Preston et al., 2000). Although dentists are likely most well prepared for the management of xerostomia, not all dental professionals receive adequate formal education on the topic (Abdelghany et al., 2011). Dentists who are more confident in their knowledge of xerostomia and the management of it were more likely to engage their patients in discussions about their symptoms and were more likely to address the symptoms in their care of the patient. This suggests value in greater preparation of dentists.

There is currently a call to educators to incorporate examinations of the oral cavity into the curriculum of a wide variety of HCPs, including physician assistants, physicians, nurses, pharmacists, and speech-language pathologists (Lygre, Kjome, Choi, & Stewart, 2017; Pogge et al., 2018; Rozas, Sadowsky, Jones, & Jeter, 2017; Yellowitz, 2016). Speech-language pathology is an often overlooked profession in the interdisciplinary oral health literature. Speech-language pathologists have a high degree of familiarity with the structures and function of the oral cavity but have not typically been trained specifically in either the assessment of xerostomia or the provision of oral care. Instead, the focus of their oral cavity evaluation for patients tends to focus on structures and function for speech production, chewing, eating, and swallowing. Speech-language pathologists will often note the condition of the oral cavity in the course of their swallowing assessment because they may be aware that xerostomia correlates with dysphagia and quality of life, partially impacted through diet choices and limitations, and also because a dry oral cavity is more likely to harbor harmful bacteria, which are likely to increase the risk of aspiration pneumonia (Husaini et al., 2014; Riquelme et al., 2008). However, speech-language pathologists are seldom prepared to focus specifically on the evaluation of xerostomia and have been given little framework in their formal education for specific mechanisms to evaluate oral health (Simpelaere, Van Nuffelen, Vanderwegen, Wouters, & De Bodt, 2016).

Although oral health assessment may be lacking in the formal curricula of HCPs, there are tools available in the form of continuing education and standardized questionnaires. Speech-language pathologists whose assessments typically include an examination of the oral cavity are well equipped to extend their observations into the realm of xerostomia. Standardized tools such as the Oral Health Assessment Tool for Dental Screening (Table 2-3) developed by the Australian Research Centre for Population Oral Health at the University of Adelaide have been shown to have been used easily and reliably by speech-language pathologists and would allow them to make a better assessment of patients' dry mouth (Simpelaere et al., 2016). This screening mechanism could easily be used by HCPs from a variety of disciplines to facilitate increased attention to the oral cavity. In addition to the OHIP-14, there are online curricular resources that are likely to be of value to those professionals who may have already completed their formal and postgraduate training and find themselves looking to improve their proficiency with oral examinations. The free web resource *Smiles for Life: A National Oral Health Curriculum* (Smiles for Life, n.d.) was originally developed by the Society of Teachers of Family Medicine Group on Oral Health and hosts materials that faculty can use for educational purposes. It also provides continuing education material free of charge for professionals. Additionally, the Oral Health Nursing Education and Practice (n.d.) website has excellent faculty tool kits, presentations, and other valuable resources to help professionals. The University of Maryland's School of Dentistry (n.d.) also hosts a list of oral health resources for the nondental professional. The current URLs for these resources are listed in the references.

Better preparation of HCPs could improve patient oral health and access to resources (Appleby et al., 2016), create a more complete view of the patient while delivering more compassionate care (Folke et al., 2008), improve collaboration across disciplines (Andersson et al., 2007), and provide a higher consistency and quality of oral care (Andersson et al., 2007; Preston et al., 2000).

Table 2-3. The Oral Health Assessment Tool for Dental Screening

Resident: _____ Room: _____ Study ID: _____

Baseline/3 months/6 months (please circle one)

SCORES

(*If score 1 or 2 for any category please arrange for a dentist to assess the resident)

Completed by: _____
Date: / /

CATEGORY	0 = healthy	1 = changes*	2 = unhealthy*	Category Scores
Lips	Smooth, pink, moist	Dry, chapped, or red at corners	Swelling or lump, white/red/ulcerated patch, bleeding/ulcerated at corners	
Tongue	Normal, moist roughness, pink	Patchy, fissured, red, coated	Patch that is red and/or white, ulcerated, swollen	
Gums and tissues	Pink, moist, smooth, no bleeding	Dry, shiny, rough, red, swollen, one ulcer/sore spot under dentures	Swollen, bleeding, ulcers, white/red patches, generalized redness under dentures	
Saliva	Moist tissues, watery and free flowing saliva	Dry, sticky tissues, little saliva present, residents think they have a dry mouth	Tissues patched and red, very little/no saliva, saliva is thick, residents think they have a dry mouth	
Natural teeth	No decayed or broken teeth/roots	1-3 decayed or broken teeth/roots	4+ decayed or broken teeth/roots or less than 4 teeth	
Dentures	No broken areas or teeth, dentures regularly worn and named	1 broken area/tooth or dentures only worn 1-2 hours daily, or dentures not named	More than 1 broken area/tooth, denture is missing or not worn, needs denture adhesive, or not named	
Oral cleanliness	Clean and no food particles or tartar in the mouth or on dentures	Food particles/tartar/plaque in 1-2 areas of the mouth or on small area of dentures	Food particles/tartar/plaque in most areas of the mouth or on most of dentures	
Dental pain	No behavioral, verbal, or physical signs of dental pain	Verbal and/or physical signs of pain, such as pulling at face, chewing lips, not eating, aggression	Physical pain signs (swelling of cheek or gum, broken teeth, ulcers), as well as verbal and/or behavioral signs (pulling at face, not eating, aggression)	

Please tick this box if the resident was referred to a dentist after screening ☐   Total score ____/16

Reprinted with permission from Chalmers, J.M., Spencer, A.J., Carter, K.D., King, P.L., & Wright, C. (2009). Caring for oral health in Australian residential care. Dental statistics and research series no. 48. Cat. no. DEN 193. Canberra: AIHW.

Figure 2-2. Common questions to begin the discussion with patients about the impact of xerostomia on their quality of life. (Adapted from Locker, D. [2003]. Dental status, xerostomia and the oral health-related quality of life of an elderly institutionalized population. *Special Care Dentist, 23*[3], 86-93 and Villa, A., Connell, C. L., & Abati, S. [2015]. Diagnosis and management of xerostomia and hyposalivation. *Therapeutics and Clinical Risk Management, 11*, 45-51. doi:2147/TCRM.S76282)

Perception
- Does your mouth feel dry?
- Do you feel that you have adequate saliva in your mouth?

Function
- Do you have difficulty speaking due to dryness?
- Do you have difficulty eating due to dryness?

Compensation
- Do you sip liquids to alleviate dryness?
- Do you use gums or mints to relieve discomfort?

Assessment of Dry Mouth/Oral Health–Related Quality of Life

As noted previously, various sets of questions, some with as few as three to five items, have been researched and found useful in identifying patient perceptions of xerostomia (Locker, 2003; Villa et al., 2015). Questions that are common across several validated questionnaires are summarized in Figure 2-2 and include inquiring about the patient's perception of oral dryness in general; oral dryness in association with specific functions, such as speaking and eating; and the use of compensatory strategies to manage oral dryness, such as sipping liquids or using gum to alleviate discomfort and/or improve function (Eisbruch et al., 2003; Fox, Busch, & Baum, 1987; Pai, Ghezzi, & Ship, 2001; Sreebny & Valdini, 1988; Thomson, Chalmers, Spencer, & Williams, 1999; van der Putten, Brand, Schols, & de Baat, 2011; Zunt, 2018).

Although the use of these questions regarding patients' perceptions, functions, and compensatory strategies do not represent a research-validated tool, they do represent categories of questions that are common across many of the best questionnaires. The use of questions across these areas may provide the HCP with the opportunity to inquire briefly and informally as to the patient's concerns regarding his or her xerostomia and its impact on his or her quality of life. From there, one of the standardized questionnaire tools should be used along with clinical evaluations, if concerns are raised. Being aware of the problem and engaging patients in discussions about how the xerostomia impacts them psychologically is a critical first step (Rydholm & Strang, 2002). HCPs must begin to engage patients in discussions about their experiences with xerostomia, rather than neglecting them (Folke et al., 2009). Dialogue with patients about dry mouth should be a routine aspect of our interactions, particularly when they have known risks for xerostomia. We must begin by asking the questions and giving patients the opportunity to talk about their experiences.

Support Systems

In order to increase the likelihood that patients are supported outside of the care that we have provided, we need to offer our patients additional resources. Patients with xerostomia cannot have all their needs met by their health care team members. HCPs can help combat the sense of isolation to improve the quality of their lives through the recommendation of support groups. Support groups, whether in person or online, can be immensely helpful for individuals who experience a deterioration of their socialization due to xerostomia (Ramirez-Sepulveda et al., 2016). Support groups can provide participants with a sense of comfort from knowing that they are not struggling with problems alone and that other people understand their difficulties. Participants in the study conducted for this text noted that online support groups were a valuable source of information and comfort, particularly in the absence of being provided with tips and tricks from their HCPs to alleviate the symptoms and suffering from xerostomia.

Patient-Centered Communication

Part of patient-centered care, as discussed in the first chapter, depends on HCPs using communication that is patient centered. Patient-centered communication is defined as "communication behaviors that can enhance the quality of the relationship between the healthcare provider and patient" (Wanzer, Booth-Butterfield, & Gruber, 2004, p. 364). Patient-centered communication increases patient satisfaction and addresses emotional needs. The use of patient-centered communication has been correlated with fewer diagnostic tests being ordered, reducing patient discomfort and anxiety, and contributing to improved overall efficiency of care (Davis, Foley, Crigger, & Brannigan, 2008; Wanzer et al., 2004). Effective communication not only aids in the development of the clinician-patient partnership, but also it can foster the desired patient outcomes (Bodie, 2014; Clark et al., 2008; Davis et al., 2008). Effective communication with patients can be learned and does not necessarily result in increased time for patient visits (Bodie, 2014; Clark et al., 2008). Communication, much like care, needs to be about the human relationship and reflect the desired back-and-forth sharing of information between the parties involved.

Active Listening

In virtually all human interactions of any importance, people want to know that they are being heard. In health care settings, patients knowing that they are being listened to is critical. It has been noted that when a physician "listened carefully" to parents of children with chronic illness, the parents were more likely to feel that their concerns decreased (Clark et al., 2008). Listening has been described by patients as being critical to several aspects of their relationship with HCPs (Jagosh, Boudreau, MacDonald, & Ingram, 2011). Patients feel that critical information in the form of their perspective is being considered when their HCPs listen effectively. Patients indicated that being listened to by their HCPs was in and of itself "healing and therapeutic," which in turn helped to reduce stress and anxiety (Jagosh et al., 2011, p. 371). Listening was observed to foster and improve the doctor–patient relationship, particularly when it is genuine.

Listening has become more critical as patients begin to take on a more active role in their health care and expect participation as a partner in their care. Patients who see themselves as active participants are likely to expect their HCPs to have more advanced communication skills (Clark et al., 2008; Davis et al., 2008). Although there are still patients who prefer to play a passive role in their health care, we are seeing more who prefer to take an active role by seeking out referrals, adjusting their own medications, and participating in decision making regarding their own care (Jagosh et al., 2011; Ngo et al., 2016).

Research has suggested that HCPs are not always good listeners. Physicians have been shown to solicit patients' reasons for a visit just over 75% of the time and to interrupt or redirect the patients' responses 82% of the time, interrupting on average 23.1 seconds into the patient's explanation (Marvel, Epstein, Flowers, & Beckman, 1999). Patients who were allowed to complete their explanation of concerns took only 6 seconds longer than those who were interrupted. One way to improve interactions is to engage in a more purposeful approach to listening. Active listening takes "courage, generosity, and patience" and can be "characterized more by what is not done than what is done" (Robertson, 2005, p. 1053). In order to engage in active listening, HCPs must withhold their own reactions and responses that may become barriers to listening well so that patients can complete the act of sharing. Thoughts and behaviors that can create obstacles to effective listening include (a) judging, in which the HCP considers a criticism, diagnosis, or evaluation prematurely; (b) suggesting solutions that include giving orders, advising, or asking excessive questions in search of a solution before the patient has finished talking; and (c) avoiding others' concerns, which is often done by giving reassurance, posing a logical argument, or diverting from the topic

(Robertson, 2005). Allowing patients the time to complete their story and then engaging with them can demonstrate that they are being actively listened to. HCP behaviors that may maximize listening include the use of more open-ended questions, particularly at the beginning of soliciting concerns, followed by more narrowly focused open-ended questions before moving to closed-ended questions (Marvel et al., 1999). This is referred to as a *funnel sequence* because the practitioner moves from broad to narrow questions (Rollin, 2000). Additionally, providing nonverbally encouraging gestures, such as head nods, and remaining silent but attentive can help give the patient a better sense of being listened to (Robertson, 2005).

Empathy

If active listening provides a baseline level of patient-centered communication, demonstrating sincere care in communication with patients will result in even greater effectiveness of communication. Insincere listening, or pretending to listen and care, is perceived to "be patronizing" (Jagosh et al, 2011, p. 373). "Caring is the gateway to disclosure" and facilitates opportunities for HCPs to truly understand what is of concern for the patient and ultimately to avoid misdiagnosing and mismanaging patients' conditions (Chochinov, 2013, p. 757). Missing opportunities for being empathetic can result in oversights into key patient symptoms. Unfortunately, in this age of high-cost health care, shortened consultation times, and larger caseloads, the pace of patient visits with HCPs can feel rushed to clinicians and patients alike. Demonstrating empathy is one way to be a more effective care provider. Patients who report that their HCPs demonstrate empathy have a greater level of trust, compliance, information sharing, satisfaction with their care, and decreased litigation for malpractice (Bodie, 2014; Chochinov, 2013; Hojat, 2009; Schrooten & de Jong, 2017; Wanzer et al., 2004).

Patients determine if HCPs are empathetic through verbal and nonverbal communication. Being attentive to the patient through the use of eye contact, facial expressions, silence, posture (e.g., leaning forward), and even laughter all convey to someone that we have empathy as we interact with them (Clark et al., 2008; Hojat, 2009). We can demonstrate verbal behaviors associated with empathy as well. Verbal behaviors that convey empathy extend beyond the use of yes/no questions, such as asking specific questions in response to patient statements, asking questions about how they are coping with life on a daily basis, and even explicitly acknowledging that you heard and understood their concerns; rephrasing what has been said in your words has been shown to improve patient perceptions of empathy and result in a more complete medical history (Clark et al., 2008; Hojat, 2009).

Although there may be differing definitions of empathy, it is important to distinguish empathy from sympathy. Empathy can be thought of as a cognitive process in which HCPs are able to consider the patient's condition and think about what it means to him or her, as opposed to sympathy, which is about sharing the feelings that the patient is experiencing as a result of the condition (Hojat, 2009). Sympathy may be thought of as "I feel your pain," whereas empathy can be thought of as "I understand your pain." Empathy as an interpersonal model has been described as including three unique skills: a willingness to see things from another person's perspective, the ability to see things from the other's perspective, and the ability to communicate to the person that you understand his or her perspective (Hojat, 2009; Schrooten & de Jong, 2017). In order for this interpersonal model to be effective, all three of the elements of empathy in Figure 2-3 need to be present.

For those who are seeking to improve their empathy, there are a number of techniques that have been shown to be effective. Hojat (2009) has written extensively on the topic of empathy in HCPs, including approaches that have been effective in enhancing the empathy of practitioners, in addition to considering the three elements of empathy from an interpersonal model as noted previously. Examples of how clinicians can develop their empathy include the following (Bodie, 2014; Hojat, 2009):

- Watching videotaped interactions with patients to practice recognizing opportunities for empathy
- Working with professional role models
- Role-playing

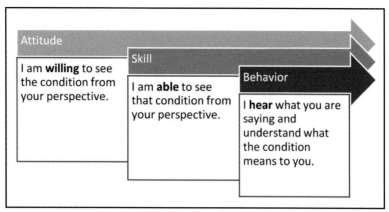

Figure 2-3. Elements of interpersonal empathy. (Adapted from Hojat, M. [2009]. Ten approaches for enhancing empathy in health and human services cultures. *Journal of Health and Human Services Administration, 31*[4], 412-450 and Schrooten, I., & de Jong, M. D. T. [2017]. If you could read my mind: The role of healthcare providers' empathetic and communicative competencies in clients' satisfaction with consultations. *Health Communication, 32*[1], 111-118. doi:10.1080/10410236.2015.1110002)

- Developing narrative skills
- Mirroring of patient behaviors, such as echoing back or adopting their posture, gestures, and speech patterns

Whether it is completed during formal educational preparation or after as continuing education, empathy skills can be improved upon and often with a lasting effect (Chochinov, 2017; Clark et al., 2008; Hojat, 2009; Schrooten & de Jong, 2017; Wanzer et al., 2004). Reflecting on the relationship HCPs have with their patients and their desire to see patients as people before they see them as patients and considering their own feelings about health care are also valuable in helping HCPs connect with why they chose their field in the first place (Chochinov, 2017). Educational materials, in the form of free online videos as a place to start, are available. What is most critical is being willing to ask patients about their condition, actively listening to their responses, and beginning to reflect on and consider paths toward increased empathy for our patients.

REFERENCES

Abdelghany, A., Nolan, A., & Freeman, R. (2011). Treating patients with dry mouth: General dental practitioners' knowledge, attitudes and clinical management. *British Dental Journal, 211*(10), E21. doi:10.1038/sj.bdj.2011.966

Andersson, K., Furhoff, A., Nordenram, G., & Wardh, I. (2007). "Oral health is not my department." Perceptions of elderly patients' oral health by general medicine practitioner in primary health care centres: A qualitative interview study. *Scandinavian Journal of Caring Science, 21*(1), 126-133.

Appleby, N. J., Temple-Smith, M. J., Stacey, M. A., Bailey, D. L., & Deveny, E. M. (2016). General practitioners' knowledge and management of dry mouth—A qualitative study. *Australian Family Physician, 45*(12), 902-906.

Bodie, G. D. (2014). Listening in health care interactions. In T. L. Thompson (Ed.), *Encyclopedia of health communication* (pp. 777-779). Thousand Oaks, CA: Sage.

Boynes, S. G., Lauer, A., Deutchman, M., & Martin, A. B. An assessment of participant-described interprofessional oral health referral systems across rurality. Journal of Rural Health, 33, 427-437. doi:10.1111/jrh.12274

Chochinov, H. M. (2013). Dignity in care: Time to take action. *Journal of Pain and Symptom Management, 46*(5), 756-759. doi:10.1016/j.jpainsymman.2013.08.004

Clark, N., Cabana, M., Nan, B., Gong, M., Slish, K., Birk, N., & Kaciroti, N. (2008). The clinician-patient partnership paradigm: Outcomes associated with physician communication behavior. *Clinical Pediatrics, 47*(1), 49-57.

Davis, J., Foley, A., Crigger, N., & Branningan, M. (2008). Healthcare and listening: A relationship for caring. *International Journal of Learning, 22*(2), 168-175. doi:10.1080/1090401080217489

Denzin, N. K., & Lincoln, Y. S. (2003). *Collecting and interpreting qualitative materials.* Thousand Oaks, CA: Sage.

Dolce, M. C. (2014). Integrating oral health into professional nursing practice: An interprofessional faculty tool kit. *Journal of Professional Nursing, 30*(1), 63-71. doi:10.1016/j.profnurs.2013.06.002

Eisbruch, A., Rhodus, N., Rosenthal, D. Murphy, B., Rasch, C., Sonis, S., ... Brizel, D. (2003). How should we measure and report radiotherapy-induced xerostomia? *Radiation Oncology, 13*(3), 226-234.

Ek, K., Browall, M., Eriksson, M., & Eriksson, I. (2018). Healthcare providers' experiences of assessing and performing oral care in older adults. *International Journal of Older People Nursing, 13*(2), e12189. doi:10.1111/opn.12189

Enger, T. B., Palm, O., Garen, T., Sandvik, L., & Jensen, J. L. (2011). Oral distress in primary Sjogren's syndrome: implications for health-related quality of life. *European Journal of Oral Sciences, 119*(6), 474-480. doi:10.1111/j.1600-0722.2011.00891.x

Ferrans, C., Zerwic, J., Wilbur, J., & Larson, J. (2005). Conceptual model of health-related quality of life. *Journal of Nursing Scholarship, 37*(4), 336-347.

Folke, S., Fridlund, B., & Paulsson, G. (2008). Views of xerostomia among health care professionals: A qualitative study. *Journal of Clinical Nursing, 18,*(6), 791-798. doi:10.1111/j.1365-2702.2008.02455.x

Folke, S., Paulsson, G., Fridlund, B., & Soderfeldt, B. (2009). The subjective meaning of xerostomia—An aggravating misery. *International Journal of Qualitative Studies on Health and Well-being, 4*(4), 245-255. doi:10.3109/17482620903189476

Fox, P. C., Busch, K. A., & Baum, B. J. (1987). Subjective reports of xerostomia and objective measures of salivary gland performance. *Journal of the American Dental Association, 115*(4), 581-584.

Frydrych, A. M. (2016). Dry mouth: Xerostomia and salivary gland hypofunction. *Australian Family Physician, 45*(7), 488-492.

Guggenheimer, J., & Moore, P. (2003). Xerostomia: etiology, recognition and treatment. *Journal of the American Dental Association, 134*(1), 61.

Haber, J., Hartnett, E., Allen, K., Hallas, D., Dorsen, C., Lange-Kessler, J. ... Wholihan, D., (2015). Putting the mouth back in the head: HEENT to HEENOT. *American Journal of Public Health, 105*(3), 437-441.

Hojat, M. (2009). Ten approaches for enhancing empathy in health and human services cultures. *Journal of Health and Human Services Administration, 31*(4), 412-450.

Husaini, H., Krisciunas, G. P., Langmore, S., Mojica, J. K., Urken, M. L., Jacobson, A. S., & Lazarus, C. L. (2014). A survey of variables used by speech-language pathologists to assess function and predict functional recovery in oral cancer patients. *Dysphagia, 29*(3), 376-386. doi:10.1007/s00455-014-9520-2

Ikebe, K., Matsuda, K., Morii, K., Wada, M., Hazeyama, T., Nokubi, T., & Ettinger, R. (2007). Impact of dry mouth and hyposalivation on oral health-related quality of life of elderly Japanese. *Oral Surgery, Oral Medicine, Oral Pathology, Oral Radiology, and Endodontics, 103*(2), 216-222. doi:10.1016/j.tripleo.2005.12.001

Jagosh, J., Boudreau, D., MacDonald, S., & Ingram, L. (2011). The importance of physician listening from the patients' perspective: Enhancing diagnosis, healing, and the doctor-patient relationship. *Patient Education and Counseling, 85*(3), 369-374. doi:10.1016/j.pec.2011.01.028

Kay, E. J., & Locker, D., (1997). *Effectiveness of oral health promotion: A review.* London, United Kingdom: Health Education Authority.

Locker, D. (2003). Dental status, xerostomia and the oral health-related quality of life of an elderly institutionalized population. *Special Care Dentist, 23*(3), 86-93.

Lygre, H., Kjome, R. L. S., Choi, H., & Stewart, A. L. (2017). Dental providers and pharmacists: A call for enhanced interprofessional collaboration. *International Dental Journal, 67*, 329-331. doi:10.1111/idj.12304

Marvel, K., Epstein, R., Flowers, K., & Beckham, H. (1999). Soliciting the patient's agenda: Have we improved? *Journal of the American Medicine Association, 281*(3), 283-287.

Napenas, J., Brennan, M., & Fox, P. (2009). Diagnosis and treatment of xerostomia (dry mouth). *Odontology, 97*(2), 76-83. doi:10.1007/s10266-008-0099-7

Ngo, D. Y., Thomson, W. M., Nolan, A., & Ferguson, S. (2016). The lived experience of Sjögren's syndrome. *BMC Oral Health, 16*(7). doi:10.1186/s12903-016-0165-4

Oral Health Nursing Education and Practice. (n.d.). *Interprofessional oral health faculty toolkit.* Retrieved from http://ohnep.org/faculty-toolkit

Owens, J., Gibson, B., Periyakaruppiah, K., Baker, S., & Robinson, P. (2014). Impairment effects, disability and dry mouth: Exploring the public and private dimensions. *Health (London), 18*(5), 509-525. doi:10.1177/1363459313516137

Pai, S., Ghezzi, E. M., & Ship, J. A. (2001). Development of a visual analogue scale questionnaire for subjective assessment of salivary gland dysfunction. *Oral Surgery, Oral Medicine, Oral Pathology, Oral Radiology, and Endodontics, 91*(3), 311-316.

Pogge, E. K., Hunt, R. J., Patton, L. R., Reynolds, S. C., Davis, L. E., Storjohann, T. D., . . . Call, S. R. (2018). *A pilot study on an interprofessional course involving pharmacy and dental students in a dental clinic.* American Journal of Pharmaceutical Education, 82*(3), 6361-223. doi:10.5688/ajpe6361

Preston, A. J., Punekar, S., & Gosney, M. A. (2000). Oral care of elderly patients: Nurses' knowledge and views. *Postgraduate Medical Journal, 76*, 89-91.

Ramirez-Sepulveda, K., Murillo-Pedrozo, A., Zuluaga-Villegas, D., Vasco-Grajales, K., Posada-Lopez, A., & Agudelo-Suarez, A. A. (2016). Perceptions of patients with xerostomia about quality of life, general and oral health: A qualitative study. *Global Journal of Health Science, 8*(11), 257-269. doi:10.5539/gjhs.v8n11p257

Riquelme, L. F., Soyfer, A., Engleman, J., Palma, G. L., Stein, L., & Chao, J. L. (2008). Understanding oropharyngeal dysphagia. *Home Health Care Management & Practice, 20*(6), 462-473. doi:10.1177/1084822308181178

Robertson, K. (2005). Active listening: More than just paying attention. *Australian Family Physician, 34*(12), 1053-1055.

Rogus-Pulia, N. M., & Logemann, J. A. (2011). Effects of reduced saliva production on swallowing in patients with Sjögren's syndrome. *Dysphagia, 26*(3), 295-303. doi:10.1007/s00455-010-9311-3

Rollin, W. J. (2000). *Counseling individuals with communication disorders: Psychodynamic and family aspects* (2nd ed.) Oxford, United Kingdom: Butterworth-Heinemann.

Rozas, N. S., Sadowsky, J. M., Jones, D. J., & Jeter, C. B. (2017). Incorporating oral health into interprofessional care teams for patients with Parkinson's disease. Parkinsonism and Related Disorders, 43, 9-14. doi:10.1016/j.parkreldis.2017.07.012

Rydholm, M., & Strang, P. (2002). Physical and psychosocial impacts of xerostomia in palliative cancer care: A qualitative interview study. *International Journal of Palliative Nursing, 8*(7), 318-323.

Schrooten, I., & de Jong, M. D. T. (2017). If you could read my mind: The role of healthcare providers' empathetic and communicative competencies in clients' satisfaction with consultations. *Health Communication, 32*(1), 111-118. doi: 10.1080/10410236.2015.1110002

Simpelaere, I. S., Van Nuffelen, G., Vanderwegen, J., Wouters, K., & De Bodt, M. (2016). Oral health screening: Feasibility and reliability of the oral health assessment tool as used by speech pathologists. *International Dental Journal, 66*(3), 178-189. doi:10.1111/idj.12220

Slade, G. D. (1997). Derivation and validation of a short-form oral health impact profile. *Community Dental Oral Epidemiology, 25*, 284-290.

Slade, G. D., & Spencer, A. J. (1994). Development and evaluation of the oral health impact profile. *Community Dental Health, 11*(1), 3-11.

Smiles for Life (n.d.). *Smiles for Life: A National Oral Health Curriculum* (3rd ed.). Retrieved from https://smilesforlifeoralhealth.org/buildcontent.aspx?tut=555&pagekey=62948&cbreceipt=0

Sreebny, L. M., & Valdini, A. (1988). Xerostomia part 1: Relationship to other oral symptoms and salivary gland hypofunction. *Oral Surgery, Oral Medicine, Oral Pathology, Oral Radiology, and Endodontics, 66*(4), 451-458.

Tanner, K., Pierce, J. L., Merrill, R. M., Miller, K. L., Kendall, K. A., & Roy, N. (2015). The quality of life burden associated with voice disorders in Sjögren's syndrome. *Annals of Otology, Rhinology, and Laryngology, 124*, 721-727.

Thomson, W. M., Chalmers, J. M., Spencer, A. J., & Williams, S. M. (1999). The xerostomia inventory: A multi-item approach to measuring dry mouth. *Community Dental Health, 16*(1), 12-17.

Thomson, W., Lawrence, H., Broadbent, J., & Poulton, R. (2006). The impact of xerostomia on oral-health-related quality of life among younger adults. *Health and Quality of Life Outcomes, 4*, 86. doi:10.1186/1477-7525-4-86

University of Maryland School of Dentistry. (n.d.). *Oral health resources for the non-dental professional.* Retrieved from https://guides.hshsl.umaryland.edu/c.php?g=94000&p=3707793

van der Putten, G. J., Brand, H. S., Schols, J. M., & de Baat, C. (2011). The diagnostic suitability of a xerostomia questionnaire and the association of xerostomia, hyposalivation, and medication use in a group of nursing home residents. *Clinical Oral Investigations, 15*(2), 185-192.

Villa, A., Connell, C. L., & Abati, S. (2015). Diagnosis and management of xerostomia and hyposalivation. *Therapeutics and Clinical Risk Management, 11*, 45-51. doi:2147/TCRM.S76282

Wanzer, M., Booth-Butterfield, M., & Gruber, K. (2004). Perceptions of health care providers' communication: Relationships between patient-centered communication and satisfaction. *Health Communications, 16*(3), 363-384. doi:10.1207/ S15327027HC1603_6

Wilson, I., & Cleary, P. (1995). Linking clinical variables with health-related quality of life. *Journal of the American Medical Association, 273*(1), 59-65.

World Health Organization. (2002). *Towards a common language for functioning, disability and health.* Retrieved from https://www.who.int/classifications/icf/icfbeginnersguide.pdf?ua=1

Yellowitz, J. A., (2016). Building the ideal interdisciplinary team to address oral health. *Journal of the American Society on Aging, 40*(6), 60-65.

Zunt, S. L. (2018). Xerostomia/salivary gland hypofunction: Diagnosis and management. *Compendium, 39*(6), 365-370.

3

THE SCIENCE OF SALIVA

Yusuf Dundar, MD; Joseph Murray, PhD, CCC-SLP, BCS-S;
Rebecca H. Affoo, PhD, CCC-SLP, SLP(C), Reg. CASLPO;
Sharon Ingersoll, PharmD; and Jeffrey M. Hotaling, MD

Saliva has multiple functions, including lubrication, a buffer effect to protect digestive tract mucosa and teeth, modulation of oral microbial flora, and antibacterial and antiviral functions. Saliva also plays an important role for proper protection and functioning of the digestive tract and the overall human body. Saliva has a complex mixture of electrolytes, and its secretion is tightly modulated by multiple factors. Oversecretion or impaired secretion of saliva may cause myriad health problems, and the guiding treatment principle of salivary gland dysfunction depends on the underlying conditions. This chapter provides a detailed discussion of various aspects of salivary gland function and physiology, as well as common salivary gland diseases.

SALIVARY GLANDS

There are three pairs of major salivary glands (Figure 3-1): the parotid, submandibular, and sublingual glands. In addition, there are approximately 600 to 1000 minor salivary glands that are distributed throughout the upper aerodigestive tract that produce secretions (Mednieks, Lin, & Hand, 2008).

The salivary glands originate from oral ectoderm into the surrounding mesenchyme during the sixth to eighth week of embryologic life (Carlson, 2000). The parotid gland is the first major salivary gland to develop, followed by the submandibular and sublingual glands. The parotid gland has unique features related to its embryologic development. The epithelial buds of the parotid glands branch and extend between the divisions of the facial nerve, eventually surrounding the facial nerve (Cannon, Replogle, & Schenk, 2004; Carlson, 2000). The other unique feature of the parotid gland is its encapsulation pattern. Although all three pairs of the major salivary glands become encapsulated, the parotid gland is the first to develop but actually the last to become encapsulated; the lymphatic

Ginsberg, S. M. (Ed.).
*Xerostomia: An Interdisciplinary Approach
to Managing Dry Mouth* (pp. 29-40).
© 2020 Taylor & Francis Group.

Figure 3-1. Major salivary glands. The illustration details the location of the major salivary glands and the associated ducts. (Reprinted with permission from Joseph Murray, PhD, CCC-SLP, BCS-S.)

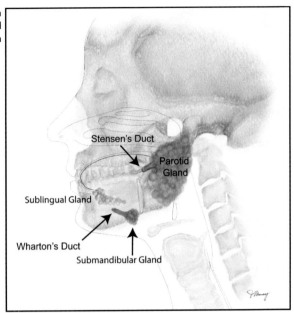

system develops before its encapsulation. This embryologic feature explains why the parotid gland has intraglandular lymphatic channels and lymph nodes in comparison with the submandibular and sublingual glands, which contain no lymphatics.

The parotid gland is the largest major salivary gland, weighing an average of 25 g on each side. The parotid gland is located in the parotid bed, which is bound superiorly by the zygomatic arch, inferiorly by the styloid muscles and the posterior belly of the digastric muscle, posteriorly by the external auditory canal and sternocleidomastoid muscle, anteriorly by the masseter muscle, and medially by the parapharyngeal space (Holsinger & Bui, 2007). The parotid space includes not only the parotid gland but also the parotid lymphatics, blood vessels, and multiple nerves. The main parotid duct (Stensen's duct) runs parallel to the zygomatic arch and pierces the buccinator muscle to enter the oral cavity at the level of the second maxillary molar tooth. Stensen's duct is approximately 4 to 6 cm in length and 0.5 to 1.4 mm in width, with the narrowest portion located at the ostium into the oral cavity (Zenk, Hosemann, & Iro, 1998). The parotid glands produce serous (thin) salivary secretions.

The submandibular glands are the second largest major salivary glands with an average weight of 15 g (Holsinger & Bui, 2007). The submandibular gland is located in the submandibular triangle bound by the mandibular ramus and the anterior and posterior bellies of the digastric muscle (Dundar, Mandle, Raza, Lin, Cramer, & Hotaling, 2019). The submandibular gland has a C-shaped form with its deep portion lying deep to the mylohyoid muscle. The submandibular duct (Wharton's duct) is approximately 5 cm in length and 0.5 to 1.5 mm in width (Zenk et al., 1998). Wharton's duct originates at the medial aspect of the gland and runs between the hypoglossal and lingual nerves. The submandibular glands produce mixed (serous and mucinous) secretions.

The sublingual glands are the smallest major salivary glands and are located in the sublingual space, which is bound by the mylohyoid, geniohyoid, and genioglossus muscles. The sublingual space includes the sublingual glands, the hypoglossal nerve, the lingual nerve and artery, and Wharton's duct. Unlike the parotid and submandibular glands, the sublingual gland does not have a major duct. Rather, it has 8 to 20 small ducts (ducts of Rivinus) that drain through the sublingual sulcus. The sublingual glands produce mucinous secretions.

In addition to oral cavity subsites, minor salivary glands can be found in the superior pole of the palatine tonsil (Weber's gland), the base of the tongue (von Ebner's gland), the larynx, the trachea, the bronchi, and the paranasal sinuses. Each minor salivary gland has its own duct to drain secretions.

Salivary glands contain acinar cells, which are secretory units. There are three type of acinar cells: serous cells (spherical and protein secreting), mucous cells (tubular and mucin secreting), and mixed cells (Ross, Kaye, & Pawlina, 2003). Each secretory unit has an acinus, a ductal system, and myoepithelial cells. The acinar cells are responsible for saliva production, and the type of the acinar cell reflects the type of secretion; contractile cells (myoepithelial cells) move secretory products toward the secretory duct.

Basic Principles of Salivary Gland Secretion

The major salivary glands produce approximately 90% of the 1000 to 1500 mL of saliva that is produced throughout the day. There are three types of salivary secretion: spontaneous, resting, and stimulated secretion. The minor salivary glands spontaneously secrete saliva in the absence of exogenous stimuli; however, these glands are innervated, and secretion rates increase in response to afferent stimuli (Emmelin & Holmberg, 1967). Resting and stimulated salivary secretions are nerve-mediated reflexes (Proctor & Carpenter, 2007). Glandular saliva is secreted in response to neurotransmitter stimulation from innervating sympathetic and parasympathetic nerves. The minor salivary glands function continuously day and night during wake and sleep (Eliasson & Carlén, 2010). In contrast, the major salivary glands secrete in response to low-grade mechanical stimulation associated with movements of the tongue and lips. They also secrete in response to mucosal dryness to lubricate and protect the oral cavity (Baum, 1987; Ekstrom, Khosravani, Castagnola, & Messana, 2012). Although the major salivary gland basal or resting secretion is produced in response to nervous system activity, it is known as the *unstimulated salivary flow rate* (Ekberg, 2012; Ekstrom et al., 2012). Approximately 75% of unstimulated whole saliva is derived from the submandibular/sublingual glands, about 15% to 20% is from the parotid, and 5% to 8% is from the minor salivary glands (Edgar, 1992; Humphrey & Williamson, 2001; Sreebny, 2000). At mealtimes, in response to taste, smell, visual, and mechanical stimuli, salivary flow rates increase by 5 to 50 times. The percentage contribution from the parotid gland increases to more than 50% of the total salivary secretions. This increased flow rate is referred to as the *stimulated salivary flow rate*. Salivary flow rates vary greatly across individuals under both unstimulated and stimulated conditions. However, a salivary flow rate greater than 0.1 mL/min is considered normal during unstimulated, or resting, conditions. Under stimulated conditions, salivary flow rates increase, and greater than 0.2 mL/min is regarded as normal (Humphrey & Williamson, 2001). The submandibular and sublingual glands contribute greatly to the unstimulated salivary flow rate, with the submandibular glands contributing 65% and the sublingual glands contributing 7% to 8% of the total salivary secretions. Additionally, the parotid glands contribute 20%, whereas the minor salivary glands are responsible for producing less than 10% of the salivary secretions during resting conditions. In response to stimulation, the flow rate from the parotid glands increases and produces greater than 50% of the salivary secretions (Humphrey & Williamson, 2001).

Table 3-1. Composition of Saliva	
ORGANIC CONSTITUENTS	**INORGANIC CONSTITUENTS**
• Amino acids • Protein • Glucose • Cholesterol • Lipids • Urea • Ammonia • Uric acid	• Sodium (Na^+) • Potassium (K^+) • Calcium (Ca^{++}) • Magnesium (Mg^{++}) • Chloride (Cl^-) • Bicarbonate (HCO_3)

COMPOSITION OF SALIVA

Saliva contains a complex mixture of electrolytes and macromolecules in which the vast majority (99%) of that volume is water, and less than 1% is composed of proteins and salts (Table 3-1). The initial secretion of the acinus is an isotonic solution. In contrast to acinar cells, ductal cells are water impermeable where sodium and chloride ions are absorbed in the duct cells and potassium and bicarbonate are secreted in the lumen. Saliva is usually a hypotonic composition (25 milliequivalent [mEq]/L NaCl) when it enters the oral cavity. The electrolyte composition of saliva is strictly associated with the salivary flow rates. There is a positive correlation between increased salivary flow rates and increased salivary sodium chloride concentrations. Another constituent of saliva is an exudate called *gingival crevicular fluid* (Sreebny & Vissink, 2010). The combination of all of these fluids, as well as oral bacteria and their products, is referred to as *whole saliva*. Physical stimulation of the glands, circadian rhythms, and age affect the type and volume of proteins and other nonwater components in whole mouth saliva. The major salivary glands are also the principal source of antimicrobial substances (immunoglobulin [Ig] A, IgG, IgM, lactoferrin, lysozyme, and peroxidases).

FUNCTIONS OF SALIVA

Saliva has five major functions: (a) lubrication, (b) buffering, (c) antibacterial and antiviral activities, (d) maintenance of tooth integrity, and (e) taste and digestion (Humphrey & Williamson, 2001). Each of these functions is discussed in the following sections.

Lubrication

Lubrication is one of the most important functions of saliva. Saliva creates a protective barrier against irritants, chemical agents, and proteolytic and hydrolytic enzymes. Lubrication is necessary for many oral/oropharyngeal functions such as speech, swallowing, and mastication (Hatton, Loomis, Levine, & Tabak, 1985). Mucin, which is secreted from all of the glands, plays a key role in lubrication (Tabak, 1995). The secretions rich in mucins have the ability to not only lubricate but also to stretch and bond to one another to form tangled grids or webs known as *spinnbarkeit* that coat the epithelial surfaces of the mouth and pharynx (Table 3-2). Spinnbarkeit is typically present as a thin film with a depth of 70 to 100 μm (Collins & Dawes, 1987) and is thickest on the posterior tongue and thinnest on the hard palate (Wolff & Kleinberg, 1998). The mucins forming the spinnbarkeit create a diffusion barrier along the tongue and pharynx, allowing for easier transport of food

Table 3-2. Important Salivary Molecules and Functions	
• Amylase	• Peroxidases
• Cystatins	• Carbonic anhydrases
• Histatins	• Statherins
• Mucins	• Proline-rich proteins

Adapted from Humphrey, S. P., & Williamson, R. T. (2001). A review of saliva: Normal composition, flow, and function. *Journal of Prosthetic Dentistry, 85*(2), 162-169. doi:10.1067/mpr.2001.113778

and liquid at the height of shear stresses during the acceleration of the bolus from the oral cavity to the distal pharynx. The submandibular, sublingual, and minor salivary gland secretions are dense with mucins and the most viscous and viscoelastic, whereas the parotid gland secretions are less dense with mucins and are less viscous and viscoelastic. Proline-rich polypeptides are another class of salivary glycoproteins that are found in parotid secretions. Proline-rich polypeptides contribute the lubrication effect of saliva by creating a protective barrier in the oral cavity.

Buffering

Saliva has an alkaline pH because of its composition. Bicarbonate and phosphates are the most important buffers, which neutralize acids from food and drink, as well as the acids produced by bacterial fermentation of carbohydrates (Edgar, 1992; see Table 3-2). These components not only maintain a neutral pH in the oral cavity contributing to the balance of the oral biome but also buffer acid in the esophagus and stomach as secretions are swallowed and transported there (Mandel, 1989). The concentration of bicarbonate increases with high flow rates, which further increases the buffering capacity. In contrast, at low flow rates, the bicarbonate level and buffering capacity decrease.

Antibacterial and Antiviral Activity

Saliva contains many immunologic mediators, such as IgA, IgG, and IgM, to prevent infections. In addition to immunologic mediators, saliva has lots of non–immune-mediated agents that help to protect digestive mucosa. Some of the non–immune-mediated components are (a) mucin, (b) enzymes (i.e., lysozyme, peroxidase, and lactoferrin), and (c) proteins (i.e., amylase, statherin, histatin, and proline-rich proteins) (see Table 3-2).

Maintenance of Tooth Integrity

Saliva plays an important role in the mineralization and demineralization processes of teeth. Demineralization is triggered by acidic flora, which is related to plaque and the pellicle formations of enamel. The optimal pH for demineralization is 5 to 5.5. The buffering function of saliva neutralizes the pH and prevents dental caries (Humphrey & Williamson, 2001). In addition to preventing demineralization, saliva helps the remineralization process by replacing minerals of the enamel. This function of saliva is further expanded on in Chapter 5.

Taste and Digestion

The role of saliva in the process of mastication, swallowing, and taste is complex and very crucial for oral functions. Amylase is the main enzyme that initiates the digestion of carbohydrates (Matuso, 2000). The main role of saliva in taste is solubilizing and transporting the ingested food particles to taste receptors. The relationship between saliva and taste is further discussed in Chapter 6.

REGULATION OF SALIVARY SECRETION

The oral tissues are among the most richly innervated of any in the human body in terms of the number and variety of peripheral receptors that they contain (Haggard & de Boer, 2014). Both slowly and rapidly adapting sensory receptors in the tongue, periodontal ligament, gingiva, and palate convey an extensive range of sensory information including touch, pressure, vibration, proprioception, pain, and temperature (Dong, Shiwaku, Kawakami, & Chudler, 1993; Nordin & Hagbarth, 1989; Trulsson & Johansson, 2002).

Information from mechanical afferent stimulation associated with oral rest conditions, such as contact between different surfaces in the mouth, and stimulated conditions, such as mastication, is conveyed by the sensory branches of the trigeminal and glossopharyngeal cranial nerves to the trigeminal sensory nuclei within the medulla. The salivatory nuclei are also located in the medulla and receive central information from areas of the brain, such as the hypothalamus, as well as the incoming sensory information from the periphery. The superior salivatory nucleus contains the preganglionic autonomic motor neurons of the facial nerve, which sends secretomotor input to the submandibular, sublingual, and minor salivary glands, whereas the inferior salivatory nucleus contains the preganglionic autonomic motor neurons of the glossopharyngeal nerve, which sends secretomotor input to the parotid glands (Wilson-Pauwels, Stewart, Akesson, & Spacey, 2010). In response to the sensory stimuli, efferent parasympathetic and sympathetic secretomotor nerves conduct excitatory signals to the salivary glands, resulting in secretion (Proctor & Carpenter, 2007).

Mastication stimulates saliva production. As the teeth move, they activate mechanoreceptors of the periodontal ligaments, initiating a short loop reflex to the major salivary glands as depicted in Figure 3-1. When stimulated by gustatory stimulation or the activity of chewing, the parotid gland becomes more productive with more than twice the output of the submandibular glands. Stokes and Davies (2007) reported that saliva that was stimulated by chewing from the parotid gland was found to have reduced elastic properties when compared with saliva stimulated by taste and smell.

DISORDERS WITH IMPAIRED SALIVARY FUNCTION

Salivary gland dysfunctions are associated with a wide spectrum of disorders. Many systemic diseases or primary salivary gland diseases may influence salivary gland functions (Table 3-3). Diseases associated with hyposalivation are discussed in the following sections.

Hyposalivation

Oral tissue dryness is a complex issue (Figure 3-2). Hyposalivation occurs when there is a reduction in the amount of saliva produced by the salivary glands that results in rapid deterioration of oral health (Sreebny, 2000). Xerostomia refers to the subjective perception of dry mouth (Levine, 1989; Navazesh & Ship, 1983). A person may experience xerostomia with or without hyposalivation or experience hyposalivation with or without xerostomia (Han, Suarez-Durall, & Mulligan, 2015). Additionally, the degree of perceived dryness is not directly related to the severity of hyposalivation (Dawes, 1987). Hyposalivation and xerostomia span numerous clinical pathologies and are known side effects of many therapeutic agents (Sreebny, 2000). Salivary gland hypofunction can be objectively measured using sialometry (Navazesh, 1993); however, the impact of xerostomia can only be assessed through recording a person's subjective perceptions (Fox, Busch, & Baum, 1987).

A systematic review and meta-analysis of studies examining the prevalence of xerostomia and hyposalivation in the general population revealed the overall prevalence of xerostomia was estimated to be 23% and the overall prevalence of hyposalivation was estimated to be 20%. A higher prevalence of xerostomia was observed in studies conducted only with older people (Agostini et al., 2018).

Table 3-3. Diseases Associated With Impaired Salivary Functions

PRIMARY SALIVARY GLAND RELATED	SYSTEMIC OR EXOGENOUS SOURCES
• Suppurative sialadenitis • Viral infections • Granulomatous infections of salivary glands • Sialolithiasis • Sialadenosis • Trauma • Neoplasias of salivary glands	• Dehydration • Sjögren's syndrome • Scleroderma • Systemic sclerosis • Cystic fibrosis • Systemic lupus erythematosus • Sarcoidosis • Rheumatoid arthritis • Diabetes mellitus • Alzheimer's disease • Chemotherapy • Radiation therapy

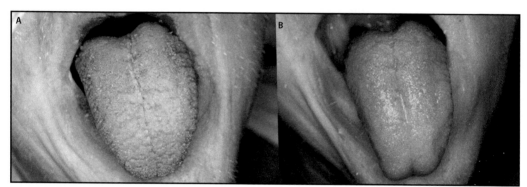

Figure 3-2. A typical view of a dry mouth. (A) A patient was admitted with multiple medical problems including dehydration. (B) The patient was rehydrated with return to appropriate salivary flow. (Reprinted with permission from Joseph Murray, PhD, CCC-SLP, BCS-S.)

Salivary flow rates vary greatly across individuals under both unstimulated and stimulated conditions. Hyposalivation is classified as a salivary flow rate that is less than 0.1 mL/min at rest or less than 0.7 mL/min under stimulated conditions (Saleh, Figueiredo, Cherubini, & Salum, 2014).

Another complicating factor that contributes to the perception of oral dryness in older adults is the greater potential for polypharmacy (Barbe et al., 2018). Salivary flow rates have been found to be significantly reduced in older adults on even a single medication known to induce xerostomia compared with age-matched control subjects (Shetty, Bhowmick, Castelino, & Babu, 2012). The reported prevalence of xerostomia for those taking medications is approximately 8% among patients on cardiovascular medications (Habbab, Moles, & Porter, 2010) to 35% in patients on antiretroviral therapy (Hasan et al., 1985), 50% in patients taking antihypertensives (Nonzee, Manopatanakul, & Khovidhunkit, 2012), and up to 71% in patients taking different types of antidepressants (Hunter & Wilson, 1995). See Chapter 8 for an extensive discussion of the relationship between saliva and medication.

Decreased salivary flow, or hyposalivation, results in profound deterioration of oral homeostasis. Increased susceptibility to dental caries and infections, decreased regulation and control of the oral microflora, and impaired swallowing may occur (Sreebny & Vissink, 2010). Salivary gland hypofunction can be caused by developmental or congenital disorders (Eveson, 2008), increased medication usage (Sreebny & Schwartz, 1997), systemic disorders, such as Sjögren's syndrome (Fox, Stern, & Michelson, 2000), radiotherapy-induced damage to salivary acinar tissue (Henson, Inglehart, Eisbruch, & Ship, 2001), and anxiety (Bergdahl & Bergdahl, 2000) (see Table 3-3). Additionally, age-related decreases of whole and submandibular/sublingual salivary flow rates have been reported (Affoo, Foley, Garrick, Siqueira, & Martin, 2015), and decreases of submandibular/sublingual and parotid salivary gland flow rates have been reported in the context of certain diseases, such as Alzheimer's disease (Ship, DeCarli, Friedland, & Baum 1990; Ship & Puckett, 1994). As discussed previously, hyposalivation does not always result in xerostomia, and xerostomia does not always occur in individuals with hyposalivation. The following discussion includes conditions in which hyposalivation and/or xerostomia are commonly reported as associated symptoms.

Radiation Exposure

Radiation-induced xerostomia affects 30,000 to 50,000 patients in the United States annually (Nagler, 2003; Sullivan, Haddad, Tishler, Mahadevan, & Krane, 2005). Radiation-induced xerostomia is strongly associated with the radiation dose/method and field of the received radiation. External beam radiation induces cell lysis in both serous and mucinous acinar cells (Nagler, 2003). Acute inflammatory reactions occur in salivary glands that are correlated with purulent exudate within the duct and parenchyma followed by complete destruction of acini cells and subsequent atrophy in the gland. Radioactive iodine can also cause xerostomia similar to external beam radiation. Radioactive iodine–induced sialadenitis is dose dependent, and parotid glands are affected more frequently than submandibular glands (Caglar, Tuncel, & Alpar, 2002).

Age-Related Decreases of Salivary Flow

An age-related 20% to 40% decrease in the volume of cells responsible for saliva secretion and a corresponding increase of fatty and fibrous tissue in the glandular area have been reported (Baum, 1987; Scott, 1977; Scott, Flower, & Burns, 1987; Sreebny, 2000). Comparable changes have been described for the labial minor glands (Drummond & Chisholm, 1984; Syrjänen, 1984). This evidence of age-related salivary gland degeneration suggests that functional reductions of salivary flow may also occur. A meta-analysis examining the effect of age on salivary flow rates revealed a significant difference between the whole and submandibular/sublingual salivary flow rates of older and younger adults. A moderate decrease of 0.168 mL/min was identified for the unstimulated whole salivary flow rate, a small decrease of 0.293 mL/min was identified for the stimulated whole salivary flow rate, a moderate decrease of 0.015 mL/min was identified for the unstimulated submandibular/sublingual salivary flow rate, and a moderate decrease of 0.040 mL/min was identified for the stimulated submandibular/sublingual salivary flow rate. The clinical relevance of the finding that whole and submandibular/sublingual salivary flow rates decrease with increasing age remains unknown. Submandibular/sublingual saliva contains mucins (primarily MUC5B and MUC7), which are much less dense in parotid saliva (Logemann, Rademaker, Pauloski, Ohmae, & Kahrilas, 1998). These mucins contribute to the oral biofilm, a slimy, viscoelastic coating of all surfaces in the oral cavity, and act as an important lubricant between opposing surfaces during such processes as mastication, swallowing, and speaking. Theoretically, age-related decreases of whole and submandibular/sublingual salivary flow rates could contribute to an increased risk of oral infection, inflammation, mechanical wear, and xerostomia as well as difficulty with speaking, mastication, and swallowing.

Neurotransmitters and Pharmacology

Both the parasympathetic (rest and digest) and sympathetic (fight or flight) divisions of the autonomic nervous system are critical to the production of saliva. The degree of response depends on the degree of stimulation. Salivary gland receptors receive neurostimulation from acetylcholine and norepinephrine, which control salivation (Proctor, 2016). Acetylcholine is the neurotransmitter responsible for sending messages from both the medulla (parasympathetic) and the thoracic-lumbar spinal cord (sympathetic) regions to the affected ganglia. Therefore, the preganglionic neurons from both the parasympathetic and the sympathetic pathways are considered cholinergic neurons. The cholinergic receptors at the ganglia are activated by nicotine and are considered nicotinic receptors (Sreebny & Schwartz, 1997).

Postganglionic neurotransmitters and receptors at the effector cells (i.e., the salivary glands) differ between the parasympathetic and sympathetic pathways. Postganglionic parasympathetic neurons are receptive to acetylcholine. The postganglionic parasympathetic cholinergic receptors are stimulated by muscarinic receptors (primarily M3 receptors with some contribution from M1 receptors; Proctor, 2016). These receptors are blocked by atropine and by other antimuscarinic drugs. Stimulation of the major salivary glands by the parasympathetic (cholinergic) nervous system results in the production of copious amounts of watery, serous saliva (Guggenheimer & Moore, 2003). Serous saliva, which is high in volume and ions but low in protein, makes up the majority of the volume of saliva. Parasympathetic stimulation also results in vasodilation of the blood vessels that support the salivary glands. Serous saliva is essential for the breakdown of the food bolus, swallowing, and digestion (Proctor, 2016).

Postganglionic sympathetic neurons are receptive to norepinephrine (noradrenaline) and are called *adrenergic neurons* at their effector cells (Sreebny & Schwartz, 1997). Stimulation of the sympathetic nervous system produces saliva that is more viscous and is high in protein content but is produced in small amounts. As a result, during periods of anxiety or stress associated with a sympathetic nervous system response, individuals may experience a sensation of dryness corresponding to the low-volume, more viscous saliva. Guggenheimer and Moore (2003) explained that sympathetic stimulation produces vasoconstriction of the blood vessels that supply the glands, reducing the rate of salivary secretion and causing glandular cells to produce more mucinous saliva. Sympathetic stimulation inhibits flow rate due to central nervous system influences from the higher centers of the brain that control the salivary centers, thereby diminishing reflex activity. This more viscous saliva results in a sticky or dry mouth feel.

There are several classes of adrenergic receptors that can be used to explain resultant xerostomia associated with some medications that impact these receptors. The stimulation of sympathetic beta receptors results in the release of salivary macromolecules (e.g., protein) with little fluid secretion. Activation of the alpha-1 adrenergic receptor results in nearly the same responses as the muscarinic receptor. Activation of the alpha-2 adrenergic receptor leads to inhibition of the actions of the alpha-1 adrenergic receptor. Higher centers of the brain also affect salivation by transmitting stimulatory or inhibitory signals to the salivary nuclei (Sreebny & Schwartz, 1997).

Saliva is an important and complex mixture of organic and inorganic constituents. Each constituent has its own function in which a small change makes a big impact on the function of saliva. The autonomic nervous system tightly modulates the secretion and constituents of saliva. Also, there are many factors that may influence the salivary gland secretions such as humoral factors, systemic diseases, medications, and aging. Subsequent chapters discuss the impact of hyposalivation and xerostomia on a variety of aspects of patient health.

References

Affoo, R. H., Foley, N., Garrick, R., Siqueira, W. L., & Martin, R. E. (2015). Meta-analysis of salivary flow rates in young and older adults. *Journal of the American Geriatric Society, 63*(10), 2142-2151. doi:10.1111/jgs.13652

Agostini, B. A., Cericato, G. O., Silveira, E. R. D., Nascimento, G. G., Costa, F. D. S., Thomson, W. M., & Demarco, F. F. (2018). How common is dry mouth? Systematic review and meta-regression analysis of prevalence estimates. *Brazilian Dental Journal, 29*(6), 606-618. doi:10.1590/0103-6440201802302

Barbe, A. G., Schmidt, P., Bussmann, M., Kunter, H., Noack, M. J., & Röhrig, G. (2018). Xerostomia and hyposalivation in orthogeriatric patients with fall history and impact on oral health-related quality of life. *Clinical Interventions in Aging, 12*(13), 1971-1979. doi:10.2147/CIA.S178370

Baum, B. J. (1987). Neurotransmitter control of secretion. *Journal of Dental Research, 66*, 628-32.

Bergdahl, M., & Bergdahl, J. (2000). Low unstimulated salivary flow and subjective oral dryness: Association with medication, anxiety, depression, and stress. *Journal of Dental Research, 79*(9), 1652-1658. doi:10.1177/00220345000790009 0301

Caglar, M., Tuncel, M., & Alpar, R. (2002). Scintigraphic evaluation of salivary gland dysfunction in patients with thyroid cancer after radioiodine treatment. *Clinical Nuclear Medicine, 27*(11), 767-771.

Cannon, C. R., Replogle, W. H., & Schenk, M. P. (2004). Facial nerve in parotidectomy: A topographical analysis. *Laryngoscope, 114*(11), 2034-2037.

Carlson, G. W. (2000). The salivary glands: Embryology, anatomy, and surgical applications. *Surgical Clinics of North America, 80*(1), 261-273.

Collins, L. M., & Dawes, C. (1987). The surface area of the adult human mouth and thickness of the salivary film covering the teeth and oral mucosa. *Journal of Dental Research, 66*(8), 1300-1302.

Dawes, C. (1987). Physiological factors affecting salivary flow rate, oral sugar clearance, and the sensation of dry mouth in man. *Journal of Dental Research, 66*, 648-653. doi:10.1177/00220345870660S107

Dong, W. K., Shiwaku, T., Kawakami, Y., & Chudler, E. H. (1993). Static and dynamic responses of periodontal ligament mechanoreceptors and intradental mechanoreceptors. *Journal of Neurophysiology, 69*(5), 1567-1582.

Drummond, J. R., & Chisholm, D. M. (1984). A qualitative and quantitative study of the ageing human labial salivary glands. *Archives of Oral Biology, 29*(2), 151-155. doi:10.1016/0003-9969(84)90120-1

Dundar, Y., Mandle, Q., Raza, S. N., Lin, H. S., Cramer, J., & Hotaling, J. M. (2019). Submandibular gland invasion by oral cavity cancers: A systematic review. *Otolaryngology-Head and Neck Surgery, 161*(2), 227-234. doi:10.1177/0194599819838475

Edgar, W. M. (1992). Saliva: Its secretion, composition, and functions. *British Dental Journal, 172*(8), 305-312.

Ekberg, O. (2012). *Dysphagia: Diagnosis and treatment.* Berlin/Heidelberg, Germany: Springer.

Ekstrom, J., Khosravani, N., Castagnola, M., & Messana, I. (2012). Saliva and the control of its secretion. In O. Ekberg (Ed.), *Dysphagia: Diagnosis and treatment.* Berlin/Heidelberg, Germany: Springer.

Eliasson, L., & Carlén. A. (2010). An update on minor salivary gland secretions. *European Journal of Oral Sciences, 118*(5), 435-442. doi:10.1111/j.1600-0722.2010.00766.x

Emmelin, N., & Holmberg, J. (1967). Impulse frequency in secretory nerves of salivary glands. *Journal of Physiology, 191*(1), 205-214.

Eveson, J. W. (2008). Xerostomia. *Periodontology 2000, 48*, 85-91. doi:10.1111/j.1600-0757.2008.00263.x

Fox, P. C., Busch, K. A., & Baum, B. J. (1987). Subjective reports of xerostomia and objective measures of salivary gland performance. *Journal of the American Dental Association, 115*(4), 581-584. doi:10.1016/S0002-8177(87)54012-0

Fox, R. I., Stern, M., & Michelson, P. (2000). Update in Sjögren syndrome. *Current Opinion in Rheumatology, 12*(5), 391-398.

Guggenheimer, J., & Moore, P. A. (2003). Xerostomia: Etiology, recognition and treatment. *Journal of the American Dental Association, 134*(1), 61-69.

Habbab, K. M., Moles, D. R., & Porter, S. R. (2010). Potential oral manifestations of cardiovascular drugs. *Oral Diseases, 16*(8), 769-773.

Haggard, P., & de Boer, L. (2014). Oral somatosensory awareness. *Neuroscience Biobehavioral Reviews, 47*, 469-484. doi:10.1016/j.neubiorev.2014.09.015

Han, P., Suarez-Durall, P., & Mulligan, R. (2015). Dry mouth: A critical topic for older adult patients. *Journal of Prosthodontic Research, 59*(1), 6-19. doi:10.1016/j.jpor.2014.11.001

Hasan, N. A., Young, B. A., Minard-Smith, A. T., Saeed, K., Li, H., Heizer, E. M., … Tabak, L. A. (1985). Masticatory lubrication. The role of carbohydrate in the lubricating property of a salivary glycoprotein-albumin complex. *Biochemical Journal, 230*(3), 817-820.

Hatton, M. N., Loomis, R. E., Levine, M. J., & Tabak, L. A. (1985). Masticatory lubrication. The role of carbohydrate in the lubricating property of a salivary glycoprotein-albumincomplex. *Bichomeical Journal, 230*(3), 817-820. doi: 10.1042/bj2300817

Henson, B. S., Inglehart, M. R., Eisbruch, A., & Ship, J. A. (2001). Preserved salivary output and xerostomia-related quality of life in head and neck cancer patients receiving parotid-sparing radiotherapy. *Oral Oncology, 37*(1), 84-93. doi:10.1016/S1368-8375(00)00063-4

Holsinger, C. F., & Bui, D. (2007). Anatomy, function, and evaluation of the salivary glands. In E. M. Myers & R. L. Ferris (Eds.), *Salivary Gland Disorders.* Heidelberg. Germany: Springer.

Humphrey, S. P., & Williamson, R. T. (2001). A review of saliva: Normal composition, flow, and function. *Journal of Prosthetic Dentistry, 85*(2), 162-169. doi:10.1067/mpr.2001.113778

Hunter, K. D., & Wilson, W. S. (1995). The effects of antidepressant drugs on salivary flow and content of sodium and potassium ions in human parotid saliva. *Archives of Oral Biology, 40*(11), 983-989.

Levine, R. S. (1989). Saliva: 3. Xerostomia—Aetiology and management. *Dental Update, 16*(5), 197-201.

Logemann, J. A., Rademaker, A. W., Pauloski, B. R., Ohmae, Y., & Kahrilas, P. J. (1998). Normal swallowing physiology as viewed by videofluoroscopy and videoendoscopy. *Folia Phoniatrica et Logopaedica, 50*(6), 311-319.

Mandel, I. D. (1989). The role of saliva in maintaining oral homeostasis. *Journal of American Dental Association, 119*(2), 298-304.

Matuso, R. (2000). Role of saliva in the maintenance of taste sensitivity. *Critical Reviews in Oral Biology & Medicine, 11*(2), 216-229.

Mednieks, M., Lin, M., & Hand, A. R. (2008). Immunocytochemical analysis of cyclic AMP receptor proteins in the developing rat parotid gland. *Archives of Oral Biology, 53*(5), 429-436. doi:10.1016/j.archoralbio.2007.11.012

Nagler, R. M. (2003). Effects of head and neck radiotherapy on major salivary glands-Animal studies and human implications. *In Vivo, 17*(4) 369-375.

Navazesh, M. (1993). Methods for collecting saliva. *Annals of the New York Academy of Sciences, 694*(20), 72-77. doi:10.1111/j.1749-6632.1993.tb18343.x

Navazesh, M., & Ship, I. I. (1983). Xerostomia: Diagnosis and treatment. *American Journal of Otolaryngology, 4*(4), 283-292. doi:10.1016/S0196-0709(83)80072-6

Nonzee, V., Manopatanakul, S., & Khovidhunkit, S. O. (2012). Xerostomia, hyposalivation and oral microbiota in patients using antihypertensive medications. *Journal of the Medical Association of Thailand, 95*(1), 96-104.

Nordin, M., & Hagbarth, K. E. (1989). Mechanoreceptive units in the human infra-orbital nerve. *Acta Physiolica Scandinavia, 135*(2), 149-161.

Proctor, G. B. (2016). The physiology of salivary secretion. *Periodontology 2000, 70*(1), 11-25. doi:10.1111/prd.12116

Proctor, G. B., & Carpenter, G. H. (2007). Regulation of salivary gland function by autonomic nerves. *Autonomic Neuroscience, 133*(1), 3-18.

Ross, M. H., Kaye, G. I., & Pawlina, W. (2003). Digestive system I: oral cavity and associated structures. In M. H. Ross, G. I. Kaye, & W. Pawlina (Eds.), *Histology: A Text and Atlas with Cell and Molecular Biology* (4th ed.). Philadelphia, PA: Lippincott Williams & Wilkins.

Saleh, J., Figueiredo, M. A., Cherubini, K., & Salum, F. G. (2014). Salivary hypofunction: An update on aetiology, diagnosis and therapeutics. *Archives of Oral Biology, 60*(2), 242-255. doi:10.1016/j.archoralbio.2014.10.004

Scott, J. (1977). A morphometric study of age changes in the histology of the ducts of human submandibular salivary glands. *Archives in Oral Biology, 22*(4), 243-249. doi:10.1016/0003-9969(77)90109-1

Scott, J., Flower, E. A., & Burns, J. (1987). A quantitative study of histological changes in the human parotid gland occurring with adult age. *Journal of Oral Pathology, 16*(10), 505-510. doi:10.1111/j.1600-0714.1987.tb00681.x

Shetty, S. R., Bhowmick, S., Castelino, R., & Babu, S. (2012). Drug induced xerostomia in elderly individuals: An institutional study. *Contemporary Clinical Dentistry, 3*(2), 173-175. doi:10.4103/0976-237X.96821

Ship, J. A., DeCarli, C., Friedland, R. P., & Baum, B. J. (1990). Diminished submandibular salivary flow in dementia of the Alzheimer type. *Journal of Gerontology, 45*(2), M61-M66. doi:10.1093/geronj/45.2.M61

Ship, J. A., & Puckett, S. A. (1994). Longitudinal study on oral health in subjects with Alzheimer's disease. *Journal of the American Geriatrics Society, 42*(1), 57-63.

Sreebny, L. M. (2000). Saliva in health and disease: An appraisal and update. *International Dental Journal, 50*(3), 140-161. doi:10.1111/j.1875-595X.2000.tb00554.x

Sreebny, L. M., & Schwartz, S. S. (1997). A reference guide to drugs and dry mouth—2nd edition. *Gerontology, 14*(1), 33-47.

Sreebny, L., & Vissink, A. (2010). *Dry mouth, the malevolent symptom: A clinical guide.* Iowa City, IA: Wiley-Blackwell.

Stokes, J. R., & Davies, G. A. (2007). Viscoelasticity of human whole saliva collected after acid and mechanical stimulation. *Biorheology, 44*(3), 141-160.

Sullivan, C. A., Haddad, R. L., Tishler, R. B., Mahadevan, A., & Krane, J. F. (2005). Chemoradiation-induced cell loss in human submandibular glands. *Laryngoscope, 115*(6), 958-964.

Syrjänen, S. (1984). Age-related changes in structure of labial minor salivary glands. *Age Ageing, 13*(3), 159-165.

Tabak, L. A. (1995). In defense of the oral cavity: Structure, biosynthesis, and function of salivary mucins. *Annual Review of Physiology, 57*(1), 547-564.

Trulsson, M., & Johansson, R. S. (2002). Orofacial mechanoreceptors in humans: Encoding characteristics and responses during natural orofacial behaviors. *Behavioural Brain Research, 135*(1-2), 27-33.

Wilson-Pauwels, L., Stewart, P. A., Akesson, E. J., & Spacey, S. D. (2010). *Cranial nerves* (3rd ed.). Raleigh, NC: People's Medical Publishing House.

Wolff, M., & Kleinberg, I. (1998). Oral mucosal wetness in hypo- and normosalivators. *Archives of Oral Biology, 43*(6), 455-462. doi:10.1016/S0003-9969(98)00022-3

Zenk, J., Hosemann, W. G., & Iro, H. (1998). Diameter of the main excretory ducts of the adult human submandibular and parotid gland: A histologic study. *Oral Surgery, Oral Medicine, Oral Pathology, and Oral Radiology, 85*(5), 576-580.

4

Causes, Evaluation, and Treatment of Xerostomia

Michael A. Blasco, MD and Jeffrey M. Hotaling, MD

Dry mouth, or xerostomia, is a common issue encountered in clinical practice. Successful management of this potentially disabling problem should include an interdisciplinary approach that should include primary care physicians, otolaryngologists, maxillofacial physicians, dentists, speech-language pathologists, and pharmacists.

Xerostomia is the subjective experience of mouth dryness, and patients may report this sensation due to either diminished quantity of saliva (hyposalivation) or altered quality of saliva. The usual quantity of saliva produced daily varies from patient to patient but averages about 500 mL per 24 hours (Dawes, 1987). Regardless of individual flow rate, patients report symptomatic xerostomia if the salivary flow rate decreases by 40% to 50%; however, many patients with xerostomia may have normal salivary flow rates. The factors behind the discrepancy between symptomatic dryness and physiologic flow rates are unknown.

Xerostomia is a common problem across all patient groups. A large review of the literature analyzing cross-sectional and cohort adult populations throughout the world demonstrated a 20.8% prevalence of xerostomia, with older adults (>65 years old) showing increased rates of xerostomia at 27.2% (Agostini et al., 2018). Some data show increased prevalence of xerostomia in women, with a Swedish study of 3000 patients demonstrating significantly higher rates in women (27.3%) vs men (21.3%) (Nederfors, Isaksson, Mornstad, & Dahlof, 1997). The overall prevalence of xerostomia in the pediatric population is poorly known despite its common incidence in children with connective tissue disorders or those undergoing treatment for malignancy.

Clinical Sequelae of Xerostomia

Xerostomia often accompanies other systemic illnesses or results from a lifesaving treatment and may often be dismissed as a minor symptom by providers. However, xerostomia has been implicated as an independent risk factor for reduced quality of life in a number of conditions, including Sjögren's syndrome (Strombeck, Ekdahl, & Jacobsson, 2000) and head and neck cancer

Ginsberg, S. M. (Ed.).
Xerostomia: An Interdisciplinary Approach to Managing Dry Mouth (pp. 41-49).
© 2020 Taylor & Francis Group.

Table 4-1. Distribution of Salivary Gland Acini and Daily Volume

GLAND	ACINAR TYPE	VISCOSITY	UNSTIMULATED DAILY SALIVA
Parotid	Serous	Watery	25%
Submandibular	Mixed	Semiviscous	70%
Sublingual	Mucous	Viscous	3% to 4%
Minor	Mucous	Viscous	Trace amounts

Adapted from Humphrey, S., & Williamson, R. (2001). A review of saliva: Normal composition, flow, and function. *Journal of Prosthetic Dentistry, 85*(2), 162-169.

(Chambers, Garden, Kies, & Martin, 2004). Every attempt should be made to treat preventable causes of xerostomia and to reduce the burden of xerostomia-related symptoms in affected patients. The effects of chronic xerostomia include the following:

- Dental caries
- Gingivitis, either acute or chronic
- Dysarthria
- Dysphagia
- Dysgeusia
- Dysphonia
- Oral candidiasis
- Sialadenitis, either acute or chronic

PHYSIOLOGY

Saliva is a fluid with a complex mixture of electrolytes and proteins secreted from three pairs of major salivary glands (i.e., the parotid, submandibular, and sublingual glands) as well as the minor salivary glands lining the mucosa of the oral cavity and pharynx. Because the saliva within the oral cavity is the aggregate of saliva produced by each gland, each with different secretory characteristics that change depending on the autonomic stimulus, the composition of whole saliva is incredibly variable (Table 4-1). In general, saliva is composed of 99% water with a pH varying between 5.75 and 7.05. Saliva has a number of crucial functions, including the following:

- Lubrication for mastication and swallowing
- Enzymatic digestion of food
- Immune defense via excretion of antibodies and pH control
- Mediation of taste

The basic functional unit of salivary glands is the secretory unit, which is composed functionally and anatomically of the acinus and the secretory duct. The acinus comprises a lumen surrounded by acinar cells. The acinus is the site of all fluid generation and the majority of the protein secretion into the salivary ducts. Acini may be classified as serous, mucous, or mixed. Saliva produced from serous acini is watery, whereas saliva produced from mucous acini is viscous.

From the acinar lumen, saliva is transported to the secretory duct before emptying into the oral cavity. Ductal cells reabsorb sodium and chloride while secreting potassium, bicarbonate, and a small amount of protein into the ductal lumen. Unstimulated saliva entering the oral cavity from the secretory duct is hypotonic, with a sodium chloride concentration of 25 mEq/L (compared with the normal 140 milliequivalent [mEq]/L human blood). The electrolyte composition of saliva is affected by salivary flow rates, with decreased reabsorption and an increased salivary concentration of sodium chloride with increasing salivary flow rates. Stimulation from the parasympathetic autonomic nervous system is responsible for the increased salivary flow rate.

The protein component of saliva is secreted primarily by acinar cells and is under control of the autonomic nervous system. A large number of proteins have been isolated from saliva, with a broad array of functions including antibacterial/antiviral, pH balance, digestion, dental mineralization, and lubrication. The most prominent salivary protein is alpha-amylase, comprising 10% of the total salivary proteins. Alpha-amylase is responsible for hydrolytic breakdown of glucose bonds in long-chain starches, resulting in the end products maltose, glucose, and other oligosaccharides. Alpha-amylase also has a small antimicrobial effect. Other major salivary antimicrobial proteins include immunoglobulin A, an antibody involved in mucosal immunity, and lysozyme, an enzyme involved in lysis of bacterial cell membranes.

CAUSES

Xerostomia may be classified as either primary or secondary. *Primary xerostomia* is defined as hyposalivation caused by irreversible destruction of the secretory unit, usually by surgery, radiation, or autoimmune causes. *Secondary xerostomia* is defined as hyposalivation caused by reversible etiologies such as dehydration, sialolithiasis, or medications. However, there is considerable overlap between these categories, and some etiologies (e.g., HIV, sarcoidosis) may cause a spectrum of salivary pathologies.

Iatrogenic

By far, the most common reason for symptomatic xerostomia is polypharmacy. This is also a major confounding factor in the investigation and treatment of xerostomia because high-risk patients for oral dryness such as older adults, people with diabetes, and patients with renal failure, will also often be taking multiple medications. Please refer to Chapter 8 for an in-depth discussion of medication and its role on xerostomia.

Surgery is a rare cause of symptomatic xerostomia. With three paired major salivary glands and 500 to 1000 minor salivary glands distributed throughout the oral cavity, rarely does a patient undergo surgery that would reduce the salivary secretory reserve to the 50% threshold generally necessary for symptomatic dryness. In a study of 130 patients undergoing parotidectomy for benign tumors, about 20% of patients reported xerostomia at the 2-year follow-up, a rate similar to the general population (Wolber et al., 2018).

Radiation therapy is a common cause of xerostomia in patients with a history of head and neck cancer. The degree of xerostomia is directly related to the dose of radiation delivered to salivary tissue. Patients undergoing treatment for head and neck cancer commonly receive radiation doses of 55 to 70 Grays (Gy). Reversible damage to salivary tissue is noted after 10 Gy radiation is delivered, with doses above 26 Gy causing permanent destruction and fibrosis of salivary tissue (Sciubba & Goldenberg, 2006). Patients treated with concurrent chemotherapy in addition to radiotherapy develop more severe xerostomia. There is some compensatory hypertrophy of nonradiated salivary tissue, and patients may report some improvement in symptomatic xerostomia up to 1 year after the completion of radiotherapy. However, meaningful improvement in salivary symptoms is rare after this period (Porter, Scully, & Hegarty, 2004).

Patients whose major salivary glands are within the treatment fields of radiation develop xerostomia at a rate exceeding 80% (Hughes et al., 2000). In patients with malignancies of the salivary glands undergoing radiotherapy, this complication is unavoidable; however, patients undergoing treatment for other head and neck malignancies, such as carcinoma of the tongue, pharynx, or larynx, may receive high doses of radiation to uninvolved salivary tissue as an unintended side effect of radiation field planning. Conformal radiation techniques, such as intensity-modulated radiotherapy (IMRT), were developed in the 1990s to limit doses to noninvolved radiosensitive tissues. Many studies have validated the use of IMRT in reducing long-term xerostomia while preserving oncologic control in patients undergoing treatment for head and neck cancer (Wang & Eisbruch, 2016).

Radioactive iodine has been implicated as a cause of xerostomia in patients who have undergone treatment for thyroid cancer. Iodine 131 is given as an oral medication to ablate remnant thyroid tissue or metastatic disease in patients who have undergone thyroidectomy. Salivary injury occurs from the accumulation of radioactive iodine 131 in salivary ductal cells at concentrations 20 to 100 times higher than plasma (Van Nostrand, 2011). Acute toxicities of radioactive iodine include pain and swelling of the affected glands, whereas late effects of xerostomia and chronic sialadenitis are reported in about 40% of patients (Edmonds & Smith, 1986).

Inflammatory

Autoimmune destruction of salivary tissue is a defining feature of Sjögren's syndrome. Sjögren's syndrome is a chronic autoimmune disorder primarily affecting salivary and lacrimal tissue, resulting in the pathognomonic symptoms of xerostomia and xerophthalmia. Classically, patients report "gritty" eyes or foreign body sensation in the eye, in addition to the usual signs and symptoms of xerostomia. Chronic irritation of corneal and conjunctival epithelium from dryness is referred to as *keratoconjunctivitis sicca*. Primary Sjögren's syndrome is defined as such when the disease occurs independently of other autoimmune disorders, whereas secondary Sjögren's syndrome can occur in the setting of rheumatoid arthritis, systemic lupus erythematosus (SLE), HIV infection, hepatitis C infection, or scleroderma. Sjögren's syndrome is most commonly diagnosed in the fourth to fifth decade of life, and 90% of diagnosed patients are women (Talal, 1992).

Sjögren's syndrome is believed to arise from interactions between the patient's genetics, immune system, and environmental exposures. Patients carrying the human leukocyte antigen B8 and DR3 haplotypes (encoding genes required for production of the major histocompatibility complex) are at increased risk of developing Sjögren's syndrome (Manoussakis & Moutsopoulos, 1999). Susceptible patients are believed to be exposed to an initial event, most likely a viral infection, that provokes the immune response. This autoimmune response leads to a dense lymphocytic infiltration of salivary tissue with subsequent antibody production against salivary cells and autoimmune destruction. Patients with symptoms of Sjögren's syndrome who present with other systemic complaints of malaise, fevers, myalgias, dysphagia, and joint pain should be evaluated for other autoimmune disorders, such as SLE.

Sarcoidosis, a systemic inflammatory disorder characterized by multiorgan noncaseating granulomas, may initially present with xerostomia and painless glandular enlargement in a minority of patients (10% in one study; Drosos, Voulgari, Psychos, Tsifetaki, & Bai, 1999). These symptoms occur from the replacement of functional salivary tissue by sarcoid granulomatous tissue and fibrosis. Sarcoidosis may rarely present as uveoparotid fever (Heerfordt's syndrome) characterized by recurrent episodes of bilateral parotid swelling, uveitis, and facial nerve palsy (Vairaktaris, Vassillious, & Yapijakis, 2005).

HIV infection may result in a spectrum of salivary disorders that have been designated *HIV-associated salivary gland disease*. Broadly, HIV-associated salivary gland disease may present as either salivary hypofunction (i.e., xerostomia or Sjögren's syndrome–like illness) or as salivary gland enlargement (Meer, 2019). Salivary gland enlargement may be secondary to several causes, both benign and malignant (Table 4-2).

Table 4-2. Causes of Salivary Gland Enlargement in HIV-Associated Salivary Gland Disease

BENIGN	MALIGNANT
• Lymphoepithelial cysts • Intraglandular lymphadenopathy • Diffuse infiltrative lymphocytosis syndrome • Chronic sialadenitis	• Kaposi sarcoma • Non-Hodgkin's lymphoma

Other Causes

Burning mouth syndrome (BMS) is a disorder of unclear etiology characterized by a chronic oral burning sensation often associated with xerostomia and dysgeusia. BMS is diagnosed in a 7:1 female to male ratio, usually in the fifth to sixth decade of life (Clark, Minakuchi, & Lotaif, 2005). Objective measurements of salivary flow are inconsistent in BMS, suggesting that subjective xerostomia may be related to altered oral sensation and not true hyposalivation (Chimenos-Kustner & Marques-Soares, 2002). BMS should be carefully distinguished from identifiable secondary causes of oral burning, such as gastroesophageal reflux disease, candidiasis, gingivitis, and vitamin or mineral deficiencies.

Transient illness, such as pharyngitis and laryngitis, may result in acute xerostomia, which resolves with supportive treatment. Chronic diseases implicated in xerostomia include diabetes, chronic renal disease, hypothyroidism, amyloidosis, hemochromatosis, cystic fibrosis, and immunoglobulin G4–related inflammatory disease (Porter et al., 2004). Alcohol, tobacco, and illicit drug use may dry and irritate oral mucosa, exacerbating xerostomia. Marijuana, both smoked and ingested, has an anticholinergic effect with resultant xerostomia. The anticholinergic effect of cannabidiol is not well understood.

CLINICAL EVALUATION OF THE PATIENT WITH XEROSTOMIA

The evaluation of the xerostomia patient is often an interdisciplinary endeavor, relying on physicians (including primary care, otolaryngologists, rheumatologists, radiologists, pathologists, and oncologists), nurses, speech-language pathologists, dentists, and other health care providers (HCPs) for comprehensive treatment. The goals of evaluation include accurate diagnosis as well as identifying preventable and treatable causes.

Evaluation of the xerostomia patient begins with a thorough history and physical. Patients may present with dry mouth as a primary complaint, or it may be a secondary concern to complaints of dysphagia, dysphonia, oral or salivary gland pain, dysgeusia, halitosis, or dry eye. Many patients with salivary hypofunction report excess saliva due to thick, viscous secretions that are difficult to swallow. Patients may report difficulty swallowing solid or dry foods, such as meat and bread. A comprehensive list of any medications patients are taking should be obtained; patients commonly omit supplements or "as-needed" medications, such as anticholinergics, and should be directly prompted. In addition to general medical and surgical histories, providers should elicit detailed dental, family, and social histories. Patients may omit previous dental infections, a family member with chronic complaints of dry eyes, or social habits, such as vaping, hookah, cannabidiol ingestion, and chewing tobacco. In nearly all cases, the diagnosis and management of xerostomia relies on a thorough history rather than adjunct laboratory or radiologic testing.

Several questionnaires and scoring systems have been developed to identify patients with xerostomia. Fox, Busch, and Baum (1987) developed a simple yes-or-no questionnaire, asking patients about difficulties with chewing or the use of sialogogues; worse scores were shown to correlate to low salivary flow rates. The Radiation Therapy Oncology Group and European Organization for Research and Treatment of Cancer (n.d.) have jointly described a standardized system for grading late effects of radiotherapy, including xerostomia.

The physical examination should include a full head and neck examination. Ocular examination may demonstrate conjunctival erythema and dryness, as well as blepharitis, in patients with Sjögren's syndrome. The oral examination may reveal chapped lips, angular cheilitis, desiccated oral mucosa, or a depapillated tongue. Dental caries and gingivitis should be noted; xerostomia is particularly implicated in cervical dental caries at the junction between the gingiva and the tooth. The quality of saliva may be thick and viscous, with tenacious secretions coating mucosal surfaces. Palpation and expression of the parotid and submandibular ducts should be performed, checking for sialoliths as well as purulent discharge. With expression of these glands in the normal patient, a thin stream of saliva may be visible from the duct orifice. Palpation of the parotid, submandibular, and sublingual glands may reveal diffuse enlargement, tumors, sialoliths, tenderness, or atrophy. Examination of the submandibular and sublingual glands is facilitated by a bimanual technique, with the forefinger of one of the examiner's hands placed intraorally and the other hand placed externally. The neck should be palpated for cervical lymphadenopathy. Flexible rhinolaryngoscopy is a common tool of the otolaryngologist, rapidly evaluating the nasal cavity, pharynx, and larynx with a thin flexible fiberoptic endoscope at the patient's bedside or in the office. The endoscopist may note thick, viscous secretions on the vocal folds as well as pooling of secretions in piriform sinuses suggestive of dysphagia.

DIAGNOSTIC TOOLS

There are a broad number of laboratory and radiologic tests that may be of use in the evaluation of the patient with xerostomia. Despite this, the importance of the clinical evaluation, particularly a detailed patient history, cannot be overstated. Tests should be used as adjuncts to selectively rule out or confirm diagnoses based on a good understanding of the patient's clinical situation.

Laboratory Studies

Sialometry is the simple measurement of saliva production. It may be unstimulated or stimulated with a sialogogue or by chewing. After a period in which saliva is allowed to accumulate, the patient is asked to spit, and the volume of saliva is measured. Although this test provides some objective confirmation of hyposalivation, xerostomia symptoms poorly correlate with salivary flow, and sialometry is a seldom-performed examination outside the research laboratory.

Laboratory investigations are diverse in the diagnosis of xerostomia. A complete blood count with differential may demonstrate anemia or thrombocytosis, both nonspecific markers of systemic inflammation. White blood cell counts may be abnormal in HIV or SLE. Erythrocyte sedimentation rate and C-reactive protein counts are nonspecific markers of inflammation; they may be elevated in patients with acute or chronic infections as well as systemic inflammatory disorders such as Sjögren's syndrome and SLE.

Serum immunologic studies are of particular importance in xerostomia. Rheumatoid factor and antinuclear antibodies may be elevated in patients with Sjögren's syndrome, SLE, and rheumatoid arthritis. Elevation in anti-Ro and anti-La (also known as anti-SSA and anti-SSB) antibodies is specific for Sjögren's syndrome, with 70% to 80% of affected patients showing anti-Ro/La serum positivity. Other secondary causes of Sjögren's syndrome can be assessed via anti-Scl 70 (scleroderma), HIV, and hepatitis C viral testing and anti–double-stranded DNA testing (SLE).

Histologic analysis of salivary glandular tissue is useful in the diagnostic evaluation of Sjögren's syndrome. In patients with symptoms suggesting Sjögren's syndrome but with normal or equivocal serum immunology, minor salivary gland biopsy may document the presence of an autoimmune inflammatory process within salivary tissue. Often performed in the office with local anesthesia or under sedation, a strip of mucosa and the adjacent minor salivary glands is excised from the mucosal lower lip. Periductal and periacinar lymphocytic infiltrates are suggestive of Sjögren's syndrome.

Imaging Studies

Radiologic imaging of the salivary glands has little use in the routine evaluation of xerostomia. Inflammatory disorders, such as Sjögren's syndrome or SLE, may demonstrate fibrotic atrophy of glandular tissue on imaging, whereas diffuse glandular enlargement may be noted in HIV or lymphoma. Structural abnormalities for which imaging is invaluable, such as stones, tumors, and salivary ductal strictures, rarely cause xerostomia.

Plain radiographic films of the salivary glands may demonstrate sialolithiasis; however, 20% of submandibular stones and 40% of parotid stones are radiolucent and may be missed on plain x-ray (Som & Curtin, 2010). X-ray sialography allows for contrast-enhanced evaluation of submandibular or parotid duct anatomy. A blunt-tipped needle is used to cannulate the duct orifice, and the duct is slowly injected with a small volume of contrast under fluoroscopy. Recent data suggest sialography has poor interobserver reliability and is of questionable use in the modern diagnosis of Sjögren's syndrome (Kalk et al., 2002). Furthermore, technical difficulty, discomfort for the patient, and the wide adoption of high-resolution cross-sectional imaging techniques, such as computed tomography (CT) and magnetic resonance imaging, have made plain radiographic examination with or without contrast sialography obsolete.

CT has become the workhorse of salivary gland imaging, allowing rapid assessment of calcifications, tumors, glandular atrophy, and inflammation. Magnetic resonance imaging has excellent utility in the evaluation of salivary neoplasms due to increased soft tissue differentiation compared with CT. Magnetic resonance sialography, which is a noninvasive technique using the patient's own saliva as the contrast, has been developed to assess ductal anatomy; its use is not widespread.

TREATMENT

Successful management of the patient with xerostomia may require an interdisciplinary approach involving primary care physicians, otolaryngologists, dentists, speech-language pathologists, nurses, and other HCPs. Treatment is directed toward (a) primary prevention of xerostomia by addressing preventable causes, (b) secondary prevention of xerostomia complications, such as dental caries and sialadenitis, and (c) improvement of symptoms and quality of life in patients with xerostomia.

Lifestyle changes are crucial in the management of xerostomia. Although many patients hope for a quick fix in the form of a pill, there is no replacement for good habits, and the treating provider should take his or her time counseling the patient with xerostomia. Adequate hydration and regular sips of water are key; patients should be counseled to keep water with them throughout the day and to hydrate with the goal of routinely clear urine. This goal may be difficult to achieve in older male patients who often limit water intake to reduce nocturnal symptoms of prostate hypertrophy. Good oral hygiene, including daily brushing and regular visits to the dentist, is helpful in preventing caries and gingivitis.

Prompt consultation with appropriate specialists is important in the interdisciplinary care of the patient with xerostomia. Primary care physicians and pharmacists are essential in treating the most common cause of xerostomia—polypharmacy. High-risk medications should be identified, and the risk–benefit ratio of their chronic use carefully considered. Patients with signs and symptoms suggestive of systemic inflammatory or infectious illness should undergo appropriate laboratory studies, and referral to rheumatology or infectious disease colleagues as appropriate. Otolaryngologists and dentists are key in the diagnosis and treatment of secondary complications of xerostomia, including sialadenitis, dysphonia/dysphagia, dental caries, and gingivitis. Speech-language pathologists are critical in the counseling and treatment of patients with xerostomia-related dysphonia and dysphagia.

Pharmacological agents for the treatment of xerostomia may broadly be divided into salivary stimulants and topical salivary substitutes. Refer to Chapter 8 for further information. In general, there is no one-size-fits-all approach, and agents that are dazzlingly efficacious in one patient may be without effect in another. In addition, some patients turn to complementary and alternative medicine for symptomatic relief. Acupuncture is perhaps the most widely used and studied alternative therapy; a recent review concluded the studies supporting the use of acupuncture to be poorly designed and underpowered (Assy & Brand, 2018).

As radiation-induced xerostomia is usually irreversible, its treatment largely relies on primary prevention. Xerostomia may be prevented using IMRT techniques to spare uninvolved salivary tissue during radiotherapy, as mentioned previously. Amifostine is an intravenous agent that reduces DNA damage by free radical scavenging in tissues undergoing radiotherapy. One randomized trial of amifostine in 315 patients undergoing head and neck radiation showed reduced rates of acute xerostomia (78% vs 51%) as well as chronic xerostomia (57% vs 34%) without affecting oncologic control (Brizel & Wasserman, 2004). However, side effects of hypotension, nausea, and vomiting, as well as equivocal efficacy in other trials, have limited the widespread use of amifostine. Salivary gland transfer (SGT) has also been used to prevent radiation-induced xerostomia. Before planned radiotherapy, patients undergo surgical reimplantation of a submandibular gland to the submental region (which is spared in radiation treatment of most cancers). A meta-analysis of 177 patients suggested SGT to be highly efficacious in the prevention of radiation-induced xerostomia, with SGT patients demonstrating drastically higher rates of unstimulated (75% vs 11%) and stimulated (86% vs 8%) salivary flow rates compared with baseline (Sood et al., 2014).

Patients with a history of head and neck radiation have special dental needs and should be under the care of a dentist with experience in this patient population. Xerostomia-related dental caries and infections may have devastating complications in the setting of irradiated tissue and bone, including mandible fracture and orocutaneous fistula. Caries may be prevented by hydration and good oral hygiene, including custom-fitted fluoride dental trays, which many patients use daily for life. See Chapter 5 for further details.

Dry mouth is a common, and sometimes debilitating, symptom across many patient populations. The accurate diagnosis and successful treatment of xerostomia demands an interdisciplinary approach enlisting the skills of primary care physicians, otolaryngologists, dentists, pharmacists, speech-language pathologists, and other HCPs. Care should be directed toward prevention of xerostomia, reduction of its secondary complications, and improvement in the symptoms faced by the patient with dry mouth.

REFERENCES

Agostini, B., Cericato, G., Silveira, E., Nascimento, G., Costa, F., Thomson, W., & Demarco, F. (2018). How common is dry mouth? Systematic review and meta-regression analysis of prevalence estimates. *Brazilian Dental Journal, 29*(6), 606-618.

Assy, Z., & Brand, H. S. (2018). A systemic review of the effects of acupuncture on xerostomia and hyposalivation. *BMC Complementary and Alternative Medicine, 13*(18), 57.

Brizel, D. M., & Wasserman, T. (2004). The influence of intravenous amifostine on xerostomia and survival during radiotherapy for head and neck cancer: Two year-follow up of a prospective randomized trial. *Proceedings of the American Society of Clinical Oncology, 23*, 495.

Chambers, M. S., Garden, A. S., Kies, M. S., & Martin, J. W. (2004). Radiation-induced xerostomia in patients with head and neck cancer: Pathogenesis, impact on quality of life, and management. *Head & Neck, 26*, 796-807.

Chimenos-Kustner, E., & Marques-Soares, M. S. (2002). Burning mouth and saliva. *Medicina Oral, 7*, 244-253.

Clark, G. T., Minakuchi, H., & Lotaif, A. C. (2005). Orofacial pain and sensory disorders in the elderly. *Dental Clinics of North America, 49*, 343-362.

Dawes, C. (1987). Physiological factors affecting salivary flow rate, oral sugar clearance, and the sensation of dry mouth in man. *Journal of Dental Research, 66*, 648-653.

Drosos, A. A., Voulgari, P. V., Psychos, D. N., Tsifetaki, N., & Bai, M. (1999). Sicca syndrome in patients with sarcoidosis. *Rheumatology International, 18*(5-6), 177-180.

Edmonds, C., & Smith, T. (1986). The long-term hazards of the treatment of thyroid cancer with radioiodine. *British Journal of Radiology, 59*, 45-51.

Fox, P. C., Busch, K. A., & Baum, B. J. (1987). Subjective reports of xerostomia and objective measures of salivary gland performance. *Journal of the American Dental Association, 115*(4), 581-584.

Hughes, P., Scott, P. J., Kew, J., Cheung, D., Leung, S. F., Ahuja, A. T., & van Hasselt, C. A. (2000). Dysphagia in treated nasopharyngeal cancer. *Head & Neck, 22*(4), 393-397.

Kalk, W. W., Vissink, A., Spijkervet, F. K., Bootsma, H., Kallenberg, C. G., & Roodenburg, J. L. (2002). Sialography for diagnosing Sjögren syndrome. *Oral Surgery, Oral Medicine, Oral Pathology, and Oral Radiology, 94*(1), 131-137.

Manoussakis, M., & Moutsopoulos, M. (1999). Sjögren's syndrome. *Otolaryngology Clinics of North America, 32*, 843.

Meer, S. (2019). Human immunodeficiency virus and salivary gland pathology: An update. *Oral Surgery, Oral Medicine, Oral Pathology, and Oral Radiology, 128*(1), 52-59.

Nederfors, T., Isaksson, R., Mornstad, H., & Dahlof, C. (1997). Prevalence of perceived symptoms of dry mouth in an adult Swedish population—Relation to age, sex and pharmacotherapy. *Community Dentistry and Oral Epidemiology, 25*(3), 211-216.

Porter, S. R., Scully, C., & Hegarty, A. M. (2004). An update of the etiology and management of xerostomia. *Oral Surgery, Oral Medicine, Oral Pathology, Oral Radiology, and Endodontics, 97*(1), 28-46.

Radiation Therapy Oncology Group/European Organization for Research and Treatment of Cancer. (n.d.). *Late radiation morbidity scoring schema.* RTOG Foundation. Retrieved from https://www.rtog.org/researchassociates/adverse eventreporting/rtogeortclateradiationmorbidityscoringschema.aspx

Sciubba, J. J., & Goldenberg, D. (2006). Oral complications of radiotherapy. *Lancet Oncology, 7*(2), 175-183.

Som, P. M., & Curtin, H. D. (2010). *Head and neck imaging.* St. Louis, MO: Mosby.

Sood, A. J., Fox, N. F., O'Connell, B. P., Lovelace, T. L., Nguyen, S. A., Sharma, A. K. ... Day, T. A. (2014). Salivary gland transfer to prevent radiation-induced xerostomia: A systematic review and meta-analysis. *Oral Oncology, 50*(2), 77-83.

Strombeck, B., Ekdahl, C., & Jacobsson, L. (2000). Health-related quality of life in primary Sjögren's syndrome, rheumatoid arthritis and fibromyalgia compared to normal population data using SF-36. *Scandinavian Journal of Rheumatology, 29*, 20-28.

Talal, N. (1992). Sjögren's syndrome: Historical overview and clinical spectrum of disease. *Rheumatic Disease Clinics of North America, 18*, 507-512.

Vairaktaris, E., Vassillious, S., & Yapijakis, C. (2005). Salivary gland manifestations of sarcoidosis. *Journal of Oral and Maxillofacial Surgery, 63*, 1016-1021.

Van Nostrand, D. (2011). Sialoadenitis secondary to ^{131}I therapy for well-differentiated thyroid cancer. *Oral Diseases, 17*(2), 154-161.

Wang, X., & Eisbruch, A. (2016). IMRT for head and neck cancer: Reducing xerostomia and dysphagia. *Journal of Radiation Research, 57*(Suppl. 1), 69-75.

Wolber, P., Volk, G., Horstmann, L., Finkensiper, M., Shabli, S., Wittekindt, C ... Groshevea, B. (2018). Patient's perspective on long-term complications after superficial parotidectomy for benign lesions: Prospective analysis of a 2-year follow-up. *Clinical Otolaryngology, 43*(4), 1073-1079.

5

ORAL AND DENTAL EFFECTS OF XEROSTOMIA

Lea E. Erickson, DDS, MSPH and Bryan Trump, DDS, MS

Saliva plays a profound role as a biologic fluid produced at and delivered to the mouth with components that function to maintain the health and integrity of oral tissues. Predictable clinical findings for people with inadequate salivary function are dry and cracked lips, mucosa that adheres to fingers or tongue blades, denuded or fissured tongues, retained food debris, new dental caries (tooth decay), fungal infections, bubbly or viscous saliva, and the absence of pooling of saliva at the floor of the mouth. Patient symptoms may be the awareness of the dryness, difficulty chewing and swallowing, needing to drink water to swallow dry foods, inability to eat dry foods, altered taste, or poorly retained dentures (Friedman, 2014). With an aging population and more people at risk for xerostomia, the management of hyposalivation to prevent its potentially devastating oral effects requires a committed interdisciplinary approach.

Case: The patient is a 56-year-old woman whose function is limited by chronic pain and depression. She lives in an assisted living facility and is treated with multiple medications to manage her pain and depression. Socialization in her living environment is encouraged by congregant meals and frequent social occasions where sweet treats are served. Her oral hygiene is excellent, and she faithfully attends the dental clinic every 3 months for preventive care. She presents with tissue that appears desiccated and does not allow a gloved finger to slide easily across it, and the saliva that is visible has a slightly frothy appearance. Her gingiva is healthy, and minimal plaque is evident. Despite her efforts at maintaining oral health and the efforts of the dental clinic staff providing professional preventive care, she presents with new dental caries at almost every preventive appointment (Figure 5-1). Her case illustrates the monumental challenges of maintaining oral health in the absence of adequate salivary flow.

Ginsberg, S. M. (Ed.).
Xerostomia: An Interdisciplinary Approach to Managing Dry Mouth (pp. 51-76).
© 2020 Taylor & Francis Group.

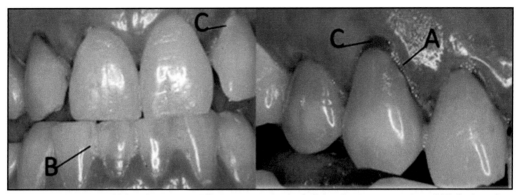

Figure 5-1. A 56-year-old female patient with severe xerostomia and the classic presentation of (A) frothy saliva, (B) multiple restorations, and (C) new caries despite good oral hygiene, daily fluoride, and regular professional preventive care.

ANATOMY OF THE DENTOALVEOLAR COMPLEX

The oral environment is an integrated system of hard and soft tissues, saliva, and a complex oral microbiome described as the sialo-microbial-dental complex (Mount, Hume, Ngo, & Wolff, 2016). Together they function to facilitate the chewing, tasting, and swallowing of food necessary for survival. When the sialo-microbial-dental complex is in homeostasis, oral health is maintained, but a shift in any one of the three increases the risk of oral diseases, including dental caries, periodontal diseases, and other oral infections. This chapter specifically addresses the role of diminished saliva on oral diseases in the context of the entire sialo-microbial-dental complex.

Saliva initiates digestion; aids in the mastication of food; facilitates speech, swallowing, and taste; and is essential to maintaining the health of oral tissues. A biofilm composed of water, salivary secretions, and microorganisms forms a semipermeable membrane that coats the teeth. In a healthy mouth, the microbial ecosystem functions symbiotically to maintain oral health. Diets high in fermentable carbohydrates and acids or alterations in the quality and quantity of saliva lead to changes in the microbiota with a resulting increased risk of dental caries and erosion (sometimes referred to as *corrosion*), oral infections, poor denture retention, and mucositis. When a diet high in sugars and acids and diminished salivary flow coexist, the disease risk is substantially magnified.

Mandible and Maxilla

The dentoalveolar complex includes the maxilla, mandible, muscles of mastication, teeth, and periodontium. The maxilla and mandible are the dento-osseous structures that support the teeth. The maxilla (upper jaw) is the fused upper bone of the jaw that has osseous articulations with other bones to form the hard palate, the floor of the nasal cavity, and much of the bony framework of the facial structure. The mandible (lower jaw) has no osseous union with cranial bones but has a movable joint that articulates bilaterally at the temporomandibular joint. The muscles of mastication create the hinge and gliding motions of the mandible that facilitate mastication, yawning, and speech (Wheeler & Ash, 1984). The alveolar processes are the portions of the mandible and maxilla that support the teeth.

Tooth Anatomy

As depicted in Figure 5-2, teeth are living organs with crowns and roots that are composed of four different tissues: enamel, dentin, cementum, and pulp. Dentin forms the majority of the mineralized structure of the crown and the root of the tooth. Enamel overlays the dentin of the crown, and cementum coats the root of the tooth. The pulp is internal to the dentin and is the one tooth tissue that is not normally mineralized.

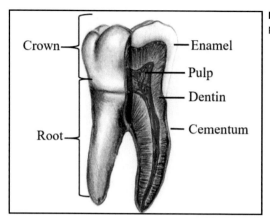

Figure 5-2. Anatomy of the tooth. (Reprinted with permission from Yuliya Petukhova.)

In its mature state, enamel is a highly mineralized tissue with a composition (by volume) of approximately 85% inorganic substance (96% to 98% by weight), 12% water, and 3% organic substance. Precursor dental epithelial cells differentiate into enamel-forming cells called *ameloblasts*. In the developing tooth, ameloblasts produce an enamel matrix into which hydroxyapatite precipitates building the crystalline structure of enamel. Although enamel is acellular, it is a dynamic structure with a flow of fluid from the pulp outward and a constant exchange of calcium, phosphate, and fluoride ions at the outer surface.

Dentin is the substructure of the tooth that supports the enamel and cementum and is approximately 70% inorganic material and 30% organic and water by weight. The border of the dentin and enamel forms the scalloped dentinoenamel junction (DEJ). Odontoblasts initiate the deposition of the matrix for dentin formation at the DEJ and progress internally toward the pulp. A dentinal tubule from the DEJ to the pulpal wall results from the incremental production of the calcified dentin. Odontoblastic processes extend from the DEJ through the dentinal tubules to their cell bodies on the pulpal wall, and tissue fluids flow from the pulp outward toward the DEJ, conferring a degree of flexibility to the tooth. The cell bodies of the odontoblasts line the pulpal wall and remain for the life of a healthy tooth, slowly producing additional thickness of dentin (secondary dentin), and, in response to chemical or microbial injury, an accelerated production of tertiary, or reparative, dentin with the resulting decrease in the size of the pulp.

Cementum is the acellular, calcified coating of the roots of teeth into which the fibers of the periodontal ligament are embedded, attaching the tooth to the bone. As the interface between the dentin and the periodontal ligament, cementum is functionally part of the periodontium. It varies in thickness and composition but is generally about 50% inorganic and 50% organic and water.

The pulp is the nonmineralized internal part of the tooth containing the cell bodies of the odontoblasts, nerves, vasculature, lymphatics, fibroblasts, and undifferentiated mesenchymal cells. In the developing tooth, the cells of the pulp produce dentin and signal the deposition of enamel. In the mature tooth, the odontoblasts respond to injury (e.g., caries, erosion, wear, dental restorations) by production of reparative dentin and by mounting an immune response to toxins from microorganisms (Walton, Torabinejad, & Fouad, 2015).

Periodontium

The periodontium, consisting of the gingiva, periodontal ligament, cementum, and alveolar bone, is the system of supporting tissues that maintains the teeth in function (Figure 5-3). The periodontal ligament is a complex connective tissue containing bundles of fibers that are embedded in the cementum of the tooth and the alveolar bone. The periodontal ligament attaches the tooth to

Figure 5-3. The periodontium. (Reprinted with permission from Yuliya Petukhova.)

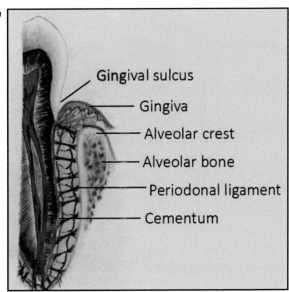

Gingival sulcus

Gingiva

Alveolar crest

Alveolar bone

Periodonal ligament

Cementum

the bone in a manner that creates a compressible sling that acts as a shock absorber and transmits biting forces to the bone. The gingival sulcus is the V-shaped trough bound on one side by the gingival epithelium and on the other by the tooth (Newman, Takei, Klokkevold, & Carranza, 2011). In healthy teeth, the sulcus will usually measure 2 to 3 mm in depth depending on the location in the mouth and the surface of the tooth.

Oral Mucosa

The oral mucosa is composed of three types of tissue. Masticatory mucosa is keratinized and covers the hard palate and gingiva. The gingiva covers the alveolar processes and surrounds the teeth. Specialized mucosa covers the dorsum of the tongue creating four types of papillae, some of which contain taste buds. The oral mucous membrane that lines the remainder of the mouth is nonkeratinized.

Salivary Glands and Saliva

Saliva is principally water (99%), which provides lavage to remove food debris, microorganisms, and desquamated cells. The submandibular, sublingual, and minor salivary glands produce saliva with mucins (principally MUC5B and MUC7) and other proteins that form a protective layer on oral tissues (Dawes et al., 2015). The salivary biomolecules and proteins that adhere to the oral soft and hard tissues interact with surface mucins to develop into a complex thin film referred to as the *pellicle*. The mucosal pellicle is initially free of bacteria (Dawes et al., 2015) and protects the soft tissues by preventing drying and providing lubrication. The acquired enamel pellicle on the tooth surface provides a reservoir of ions for remineralization, lubrication, and buffering (Hannig, Hannig, Kensche, & Carpenter, 2017). The acquired enamel pellicle develops within seconds of its removal when exposed to saliva (Dawes et al., 2015) and provides both the substrate for colonization of bacteria to develop the biofilm covering the tooth and enzymes to favor the selection of harmless bacteria (Lendenmann, Grogan, & Oppenheim, 2000). See Chapter 3 for further discussion of saliva.

Biofilm

A biofilm is a three-dimensionally organized assemblage of microorganisms and extracellular polysaccharides attached to a surface (Donlan, 2002). A healthy dental biofilm, consisting of hundreds of different species of microorganisms existing symbiotically, provides important benefits to the host, including modulating inflammatory responses, immunologic priming (Marsh, Head, & Devine, 2015), and maintaining the health of the dentition. When in balance, it acts as a semipermeable membrane that protects the tooth from wear and acidic erosion, provides a reservoir of ions necessary to maintain tooth mineralization, and buffers acids (Kaidonis & Townsend, 2016). Saliva is the source that supplies the electrolytes that buffer acids and remineralize the tooth structure. Decreased salivary flow and increased dietary carbohydrates are key factors in shifting the delicate ecological balance from a protective biofilm to a pathological plaque, one that may cause caries, gingivitis, or periodontitis.

DISEASES OF THE ORAL CAVITY

Poor Diet

Dentitions of Paleolithic hunter-gatherers showed much more wear from abrasive foods than modern dentitions, but far less evidence of erosion/corrosion and the oral diseases of caries, gingivitis, and periodontitis. With the advent of farming and, more recently, the widespread availability of fermentable carbohydrates and acidic foods and beverages, the ecosystem of the biofilm shifted to become more acidogenic with the resulting adverse effects of caries and erosion/corrosion. Many beverages, such as soft drinks, sports drinks, wine, and juices, are very acidic and often replace water for quenching thirst. In addition, they are frequently consumed for reasons beyond thirst, including enjoyment of the flavors, habit, and the belief that they have added health benefits. People commonly sip them over time, continuously bathing the biofilm in acid to create an environment that selects acidophilic bacteria in the biofilm. The role of refined carbohydrates, especially sucrose, in shifting the plaque biofilm to select aciduric (able to survive in an acidic environment) and acidogenic (acid producing) bacteria is well established, and, as with acids, the frequency of exposures to fermentable carbohydrates is an important element of its contribution to the cariogenicity (ability to produce caries) of a plaque biofilm.

Caries

Globally, untreated dental caries (tooth decay) in permanent teeth affected 2.5 million people in 2015, and remains the most prevalent disease in the world at an age-standardized rate of 34.1% of people worldwide (Kassenbaum et al., 2017). According to the Centers for Disease Control and Prevention, in 2011 to 2012, 27% of adults in the United States had untreated caries, and well over 90% have had caries experience (i.e., have either active caries lesions or restorations; Dye, Thornton-Evans, Li, & Iafolla, 2015). Dental caries is a preventable bacterial disease requiring a susceptible host (tooth), a pathological plaque biofilm, and the presence of fermentable carbohydrates. Caries is a multifactorial complex disease with the progressive loss of calcified tooth structure due to acid produced by acidogenic bacteria. A caries lesion is the clinical manifestation of the disease process along a continuum ranging from health to initial mineral loss (Figure 5-4) to moderate mineral loss to advanced mineral loss (Figure 5-5). Coronal caries begins in the highly calcified enamel and root caries (Figure 5-6) in the less calcified cementum or dentin with a resulting different pattern and speed of progression. In the initial stages, the caries lesion is noncavitated and may present with a frosty white spot appearance. Initial caries lesions are amenable to arresting the disease process and reversing the loss with remineralization. As the disease progresses, the tooth loses surface integrity and becomes cavitated, requiring a restoration to arrest the disease process (Young et al., 2015).

Figure 5-4. Initial caries. (A) Typical "white spot" lesion at the gingival margin and (B) approximal lesion on the surface just gingival to the contact with the adjacent tooth.

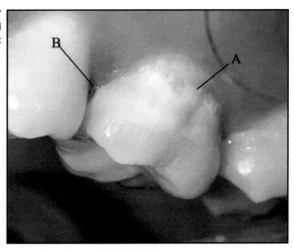

Figure 5-5. Advanced caries lesions.

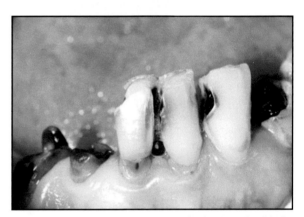

Figure 5-6. Root caries. Note the aggressive extent to the lesions in the absence of coronal (crown) caries.

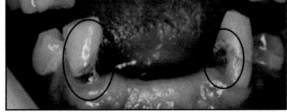

A healthy biofilm ranges from slightly acidic to slightly alkaline depending on diet and the bacterial species that comprise the biofilm. The ingestion of sugars results in acidification of the biofilm and demineralization of the tooth structure. After the sugar challenge, the buffering capacity of the biofilm returns the pH to neutral, and the calcium, phosphate, and fluoride ions that are present remineralize the tooth structure. Saliva, as the source of the minerals that remineralize the tooth structure, is critical to maintaining the calcified tooth structure (Pitts et al., 2017). In homeostasis, the cycle of demineralization and remineralization maintains healthy calcified enamel or exposed dentin and cementum, and the biofilm continues to return to a neutral pH (Figure 5-7).

If sugar challenges are frequent, the biofilm remains acidic and will select for aciduric and acidogenic bacteria, principally *Streptococcus mutans* and *Lactobacillus* groups of bacteria, but potentially including other bacteria and even *Candida albicans* (Gao, Jiang, Koh, & Hsu, 2016). The complex of organisms involved in coronal caries appears to differ from those in root caries. As the acidic biofilm

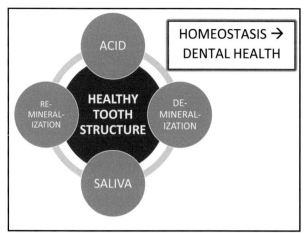

Figure 5-7. Homeostasis: A constant exchange of ions occurs between the surface of the tooth structure and the biofilm that coats the tooth. Acids produced by bacteria in dental plaque or dietary acids accelerate the loss of calcium and phosphate ions. Saliva provides ions to remineralize the tooth and buffers to neutralize the acids. In homeostasis, demineralization equals remineralization.

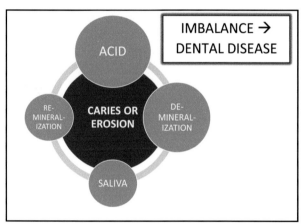

Figure 5-8. Imbalance: An increase in acids produced by bacteria in dental plaque or dietary acids or a decrease in salivary flow disrupts the equilibrium, tipping the balance toward dental caries or erosion depending on the source of the acid. The combination of both increased acid and reduced salivary flow compounds the effect of each, resulting in accelerated loss of calcified tooth structure.

outpaces its buffering capacity, the disruption of the demineralization–remineralization balance results in greater demineralization than remineralization and the consequent loss of the calcified tooth structure (Figure 5-8). The demineralization begins slightly beneath the surface of the tooth and progresses internally, eventually becoming cavitated (Featherstone, 2008; Mount et al., 2016). In the initial stage of dental caries, the disease progression can be arrested and the tooth remineralized by treatment with fluoride (and potentially other agents) and by changes in dietary and oral hygiene practices. Moderate and severe caries lesions, those that are cavitated, require restoration to control the disease and, if advanced to the pulp, may require endodontic (root canal) therapy or extraction.

Erosion/Corrosion

Dental erosion, or corrosion, is the loss of the calcified tooth structure by chemical means that are not bacterially produced. Gastric acid is the usual intrinsic source, and dietary acids are the most common extrinsic source, but other sources of extrinsic acids that may contribute to erosion/corrosion are occupational exposure, such as workers exposed to battery acid or wine tasters, and recreational exposure, such as highly chlorinated swimming pools (Kanzow, Wegehaupt, Attin, & Wiegand, 2016). People with anorexia nervosa, bulimia (Figure 5-9), and gastroesophageal reflux

Figure 5-9. Erosion/corrosion from stomach acid in a patient with bulimia. Note the exposure of (A) dentin on the entire palatal surface with (B) only a small amount of enamel remaining at the borders and (C) the pulp actually visible through the dentin in some teeth.

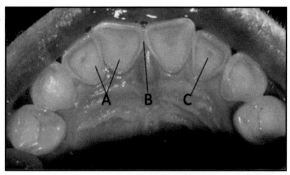

Figure 5-10. Erosion/corrosion with the typical "ditching" seen when (A) dentin is dissolved at a more rapid pace than (B) enamel. This pattern on cusp tips is commonly associated with gastroesophageal reflux disease.

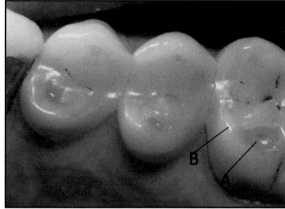

disease (Figure 5-10) have distinctive patterns of erosion, most often occurring on the palatal surfaces of the maxillary teeth and the occlusal (biting) surface of the molars. The loss of tooth structure from acidic beverages is more generalized throughout the mouth, but erosion from diet may be localized due to chewing patterns or habits associated with the food or beverage being consumed. For example, people who suck on lemons often have erosion on the facial surfaces of maxillary incisors (Buzalaf, Hannas, & Kato, 2012).

As with caries, dissolution of the tooth structure begins at the surface of the enamel or dentin. The rate and extent of erosion/corrosion are modulated by a variety of factors, including the type of acid and the frequency and duration of contact. Because dentin dissolves at a higher pH than enamel, once it is exposed, it dissolves at a faster rate than the enamel, resulting in dished out areas. Saliva plays a key protective role by diluting and clearing acids from the oral cavity, providing the mucins that establish and maintain the pellicle, and providing the ions that remineralize the calcified tooth structure (Buzalaf et al., 2012; Mount et al., 2016). The pellicle and a healthy biofilm that are established and maintained by salivary secretions are essential to preserving the balance of demineralization and remineralization that conserves the enamel and dentin (see Figure 5-7). Frequent contact with acids and/or very low pH acids may exceed the ability of the saliva and its derived biofilm to remineralize at the same pace as the demineralization is occurring with the resulting loss of calcified tooth structure. In the absence of adequate salivary flow, the body loses all defenses against acid attack with the predictable increase in the rate of erosion/corrosion (see Figure 5-8).

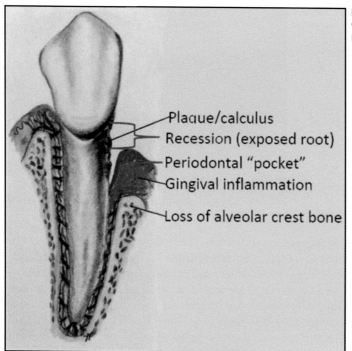

Figure 5-11. Periodontics. (Reprinted with permission from Yuliya Petukhova.)

Plaque/calculus

Recession (exposed root)

Periodontal "pocket"

Gingival inflammation

Loss of alveolar crest bone

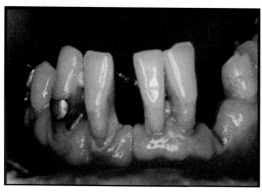

Figure 5-12. Periodontitis with advanced bone loss and recession.

Periodontal Disease

The diseases of the periodontium, gingivitis and periodontitis, are fundamentally inflammatory responses to a pathogenic biofilm in the gingival sulcus. Gingivitis is limited to the gingival tissues; is characterized by redness, swelling, and bleeding when probed with a dental instrument or during toothbrushing (Holm-Pedersen, Walls, & Ship, 2015); and is reversible. Periodontitis is similarly an inflammatory response to a complex microbial plaque, but affecting the periodontal ligament and alveolar bone, resulting in loss of their attachment (Figure 5-11). The loss of alveolar crest bone may result in the development of deep pockets if the gingival tissue does not recede with the bone or exposed roots with gingival recession (Figure 5-12). In its most severe stage, teeth become loose and are eventually lost. Chronic periodontitis is insidious with minimal symptoms until the advanced stages. The key risk factors for the continuum of periodontal diseases are genetics, smoking, type 2 diabetes, poor nutrition, stress, and, most importantly, the inflammatory response to a plaque biofilm that accumulates at the gingival margin or within the gingival sulcus (Chapple et al., 2015). Organic salivary components, like lysozyme, lactoferrin, lactoperoxidase, and histatins

Figure 5-13. Denture stomatitis. Candidal infection of the palate of denture wearers often associated with xerostomia.

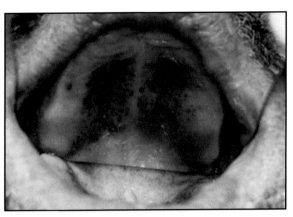

inhibit microbial growth by limiting aggregation (Friedman, 2014; Newman et al., 2011), and salivary flow dilutes and eliminates the products of the bacterial plaque. Although animal models have demonstrated increased periodontal disease with the removal of salivary glands, a protective role for saliva in humans is intuitive based on the presence of antimicrobial enzymes. Although many authors write about diminished salivary function as a risk factor for periodontal disease, evidence to support the assumed risk is minimal. However, periodontal bone loss does result in exposure of the roots of the teeth, a recognized risk factor for root caries. Because cementum and dentin dissolve at a higher pH than enamel, root caries progresses more rapidly than caries initiated in enamel. Therefore, the prevention of periodontitis is a highly relevant issue for individuals with hyposalivation independent of whether xerostomia is a direct risk factor for periodontitis. Because the prevalence of periodontal bone loss is increased in older adults (the population at greatest risk for being on medications and having diseases that cause xerostomia), the prevention of periodontal bone loss to reduce root caries risk is discussed in the caries prevention section.

Mucositis

Oral mucositis is any inflammation of the mucosa of the mouth with the classic signs of erythema, pain, and, in severe forms, ulceration and bleeding. Saliva supports the mucosal pellicle that maintains moisture in the tissues and provides lubrication, allowing ease in chewing and swallowing. In the absence of adequate lubrication, the risk of trauma from food being masticated is increased. Prostheses (dentures) depend on the mucosal pellicle and salivary film for both retention and protection from frictional trauma. In addition to poor denture retention, insufficient salivary function may contribute to the development of denture stomatitis and frank ulcers. An additional challenge for wearers of dental prostheses is an increased risk of candidiasis.

Candidiasis is the most common fungal infection in the mouth (Akpan & Morgan, 2002). It usually develops in the presence of a predisposing condition (e.g., immunodeficiency, diabetes, corticosteroid therapy, hyposalivation, poor oral hygiene). Oral candidiasis can present as erythematous or pseudomembranous plaques. Specific forms include denture stomatitis (associated with dentures) as seen in Figure 5-13 or angular cheilitis (fungal infections at the corners of the mouth) as in Figure 5-14. Hyposalivation has been identified as an independent predictor of candidiasis in subjects with Sjögren's syndrome. With normal salivary function, salivary enzymes, especially the histatins, are effective antifungal agents. The mucosal pellicle resists the adhesion and colonization of fungal colonies, and saliva washes away desquamated cells with attached fungal colonies. Candida growth is favored by the acidic environment that results from the loss of saliva's buffering capacity (Akpan & Morgan, 2002). Lesions are caused by *C albicans* or other species when the flora of the mouth is altered. The incidence of *Candida* isolated from the oral cavity is approximately 45% in children and healthy adults (Akpan & Morgan, 2002). Because of this, a positive culture in and of itself is not diagnostic; additional clinical correlation is required.

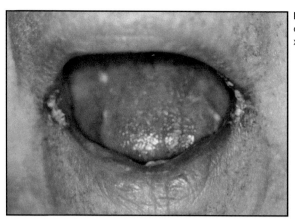

Figure 5-14. Angular cheilitis. Candidal infection of the corners of the mouth often associated with xerostomia.

CONTROLLING ORAL DISEASE

Reducing the Risk of Caries

In 1891, Dr. G. V. Black, described as the "father of operative dentistry," developed a standardized classification system for caries lesions based on their location and the type of preparation necessary for restoration of the cavitated lesion (Jain & Jain, 2017). Dr. Black's classification remained the standard for over 100 years, but as the caries disease process became better understood, the dental profession began a paradigm shift from approaching the caries from a surgical perspective to a medical model of disease management. Dr. Black presaged this change when he wrote, "The day is surely coming … when we will be engaged in practicing preventive rather than reparative dentistry" (Young et al., 2015). The concept of caries prevention is not new. The change is in recognizing disease risk or diagnosing early disease and intervening in a manner that arrests the disease and remineralizes the tooth structure rather than waiting for evidence of cavitation and placing restorations to control disease.

The development of tools to assess risk and linking effective interventions has received much attention in the past 20 years. The American Dental Association (ADA) publishes a caries risk assessment (CRA) form that has providers assess general health conditions, oral clinical conditions, and other contributing factors to determine whether the patient is at low, moderate, or high risk for caries (ADA, 2011). Featherstone and colleagues published the caries management by risk assessment (CAMBRA) philosophy and their CRA, which ranks risk as low, moderate, high, or extreme. They describe the balance/imbalance between disease indicators (i.e., evidence of past or present caries activity), risk factors (i.e., pathogenic plaque, hyposalivation, and cariogenic diet), and protective factors (e.g., saliva, fluoride, effective oral hygiene) (Featherstone et al., 2012; Young & Featherstone, 2013). The CAMBRA-CRA is a validated predictive tool for of increased caries incidence for people in all risk groups (Featherstone & Chaffee, 2018) In both the ADA risk assessment and the CAMBRA-CRA, xerostomia is a factor that automatically results in assignment to a high- or extreme-risk category.

Oral Health Maintenance

The ADA (2018) provides the following guidance for preventing dental caries:
- Brush twice per day with a fluoride toothpaste.
- Clean between teeth daily with floss or an interdental cleaner.
- Eat nutritious and balanced meals and limit snacking.
- Check with your dentist about the use of supplemental fluoride, which strengthens teeth, and about the use of dental sealants (a plastic protective coating) applied to the chewing surfaces of the back teeth (where decay often starts) to protect them from decay.
- Visit your dentist regularly for professional cleanings and oral examination.

Mechanical Plaque Disruption

The gold standard for the prevention of caries, gingivitis, and periodontitis is and has long been the disruption of the plaque biofilm by toothbrushing and interproximal cleaners (Arweiler & Netuschil, 2016), such as dental floss, interproximal brushes, wood sticks, and oral irrigators (Chapple et al., 2015). Recommendations vary from brushing after every meal to brushing twice daily to brushing daily. Some dental professionals advocate the importance of brushing at night, and others recommend brushing in the morning. Little evidence supports one opinion over another, but the importance of effective plaque removal is accepted as essential to oral health maintenance. The ADA advocates for twice daily brushing, and, independent of whether plaque control requires more than one brushing per day, the dentition benefits from more frequent applications of fluoride in toothpaste. The removal of plaque biofilm that has matured in the presence of fermentable carbohydrates and becomes cariogenic allows the establishment of a new protective biofilm with its critical metabolic, physiologic, antimicrobial, and immunologic functions (Kilian et al., 2016).

Studies to determine the true effect of toothbrushing on caries prevention have yielded equivocal results but suggest that frequent brushers have a lower incidence of new caries. In a systematic review and meta-analysis, Kumar, Tadakamadia, and Johnson (2016) stated, "It is widely believed that effective removal of dental biofilm by toothbrushing can reduce the development of new carious lesions but the evidence is weak—especially when it comes to frequency of brushing" (p. 1235). Variations in study design, populations studied, and methods to diagnose caries have resulted in limited numbers of studies that qualify for inclusion in meta-analyses. Many studies are based on self-reported brushing behaviors that may have been inflated, and reporting that brushing has occurred does not mean that plaque has been removed. The duration of brushing, the skill of the individual using the brush, and the type of brush have an impact on the effectiveness of biofilm disruption, and the type of dentifrice (fluoride vs nonfluoride) will influence the contribution to caries prevention. Whether the toothbrush is used to dislodge plaque or deliver fluoride to decrease tooth solubility and/or remineralize it, toothbrushing remains an important adjunct to caries prevention. Additionally, the mechanical removal of plaque biofilm is an effective means of reversing and preventing gingivitis (Newman et al., 2011), the first phase in the continuum of periodontal diseases, and preventing its advancement to periodontitis (Lertpimonchai, Rattanasiri, Arj-Ong Vallibhakara, Attia, & Thakkinstian, 2017). Preventing periodontal bone loss eliminates a necessary risk factor for root caries (i.e., the exposure of roots to the oral environment). Toothbrushing alone is not sufficient because the brush bristles cannot contact all surfaces of the teeth. Flossing and/or other interdental cleaners are essential for interproximal cleaning and have been shown to reduce gingivitis when added to toothbrushing compared with brushing alone (Jepsen et al., 2017). Decreased evidence of periodontal disease, less caries, and more teeth present were significantly associated with the use of interdental cleaners using data from the National Health and Nutrition Examination Survey (Marchesan et al., 2018). Some evidence suggests that interdental brushes and water-jet devices are more effective than dental floss in reducing gingivitis (Kotsakis, Lian, Ioannou, Michalowicz, John, & Chu, 2018), but they can only be used where space allows their interproximal placement without trauma (Chapple et al., 2015). Dental floss remains the primary device for cleaning between teeth to maintain gingival and periodontal health in the absence of disease, but flossing is a technically demanding oral hygiene skill. Effective flossers with a healthy periodontium should be encouraged to continue. However, in the presence of gingival inflammation or evidence of ineffective plaque removal with floss, interdental brushes or water-jet devices should be recommended (Kotsakis et al., 2018). The essential goal is to reduce plaque and control disease, so the device that is most acceptable to the patient and most effective in his or her hands should be identified and offered as an alternative.

DEVICES FOR MECHANICAL PLAQUE REMOVAL

Toothbrushes

Many brands and designs of manual and powered toothbrushes are available. The selection of a brush should largely be based on the preference of the user because efficacy depends far more on the use of the brush than the type of brush. The head of the brush should fit easily in the mouth of the user, and the handle should be comfortable to hold. Soft bristles are recommended to reduce the risk of trauma to soft tissues and abrasion to the tooth structure. Both manual and powered brushes are effective at reducing plaque if used properly (Van der Weijden & Slot, 2015). Manual brushes with flat-trim bristle designs, multilevel bristles, or crisscross designs have all been shown to reduce both plaque and gingivitis (Chapple et al., 2015). Powered brushes have demonstrated more efficacy at reduction in both plaque and gingivitis than manual brushes (Yaacob et al., 2014; Van der Weijden & Slot, 2015), and a greater reduction in plaque scores was achieved for recharge-able brushes compared with those with replaceable batteries (Chapple et al., 2015). The removal of plaque is dependent on the mechanical action of the device with no contribution from a dentifrice (Valkenburg, Slot, Bakker, & Van der Weijden, 2016). The advantages of the use of a dentifrice are to deliver fluoride, to provide an abrasive to remove extrinsic stains, and to leave a pleasant taste in the mouth. People often report that they have not brushed because they had no toothpaste, which sup-ports its use as a social norm and its value to the user as a flavoring agent. The misconception that toothpaste is essential for toothbrushing creates an opportunity for health care providers to deliver education about effective biofilm removal and to potentially affect behavior change.

Many brushing techniques have been advocated over time from a simple scrub brushing to the more complex Bass, or sulcular, brushing technique (Bass, 1954). The scrub technique is easy for children to master and is usually the first learned. For adults, and especially for high-risk patients, a more sophisticated technique is required to control disease. In 1954, Dr. Charles C. Bass, a physician whose research was in parasitology and bacteriology, published "An Effective Method of Personal Oral Hygiene" describing the sulcular toothbrushing technique that became the standard for most of the dental professions (Bass, 1954).

The sulcular brushing technique is as follows:

1. Apply a fluoride-containing dentifrice to the toothbrush.

2. Using a soft-bristled brush (manual or powered), place the bristles at a 45-degree angle into the gingival sulcus (usually covering two to three teeth) pointing toward the roots of the teeth (Figure 5-15).

3. Keeping the bristles in contact with the tooth, vibrate the brush or move in small circles for a count of 10. Some people advocate rolling the brush toward the biting surface of the tooth at this point to brush loosened plaque away from the sulcus (modified Bass technique).

Figure 5-15. Sulcular brushing (Bass technique). Soft-bristled brush at a 45-degree angle with bristles placed into the gingival sulcus and followed by vibratory or small circular movements.

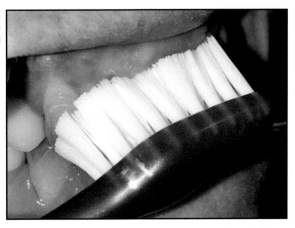

4. Move the brush to the next group of teeth and repeat systematically working around the mouth (maxilla and mandible), cheek/lip sides, and tongue/palate sides.

5. A minimum of 2 minutes should be spent brushing.

6. Expectorate without rinsing, and do not eat or drink for 30 minutes to maximize contact of the fluoride with the tooth and to increase the probability of its incorporation into the newly developing biofilm.

7. Replace brushes at least every 3 months and more often if the bristles become splayed.

Interdental Cleaners

Interdental cleaners include the following:

- Dental floss (for use to maintain health where space does not allow easy passage of interdental brushes)
  - Available in various types: Waxed, unwaxed, tufted, fine, heavier, and Gore-tex
  - Selection of type to be based on patient preference and ease of use
  - Floss holders
    - For people who lack the dexterity or physical ability to effectively use their fingers to manipulate the floss
    - Packaged with floss attached (simple and convenient)
    - Reusable handles to attach floss (easier to hold)
- Interdental brushes (highly effective in sites where space allows their placement)
  - Nylon bristles on a wire in a bottle brush arrangement
    - Cylindrical, hourglass, or tapered shapes in multiple sizes
    - Replaceable on a reusable handle or with a permanently attached handle
    - Require daily replacement
    - Available with fluoride
  - Rubber shaft with multiple fine rubber bristles radiating out from the shaft
    - Latex free by the report of at least one manufacturer
    - Single use
    - Available in multiple sizes
- Toothpicks
  - Handles available
  - Require skill to avoid damaging gingival tissues

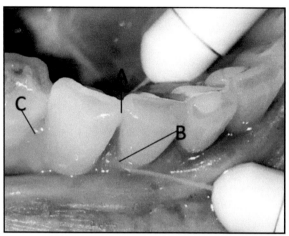

Figure 5-16. Flossing. (A) Place dental floss through the contact and gently into (B) the gingival sulcus in a C-shape. With the floss in firm contact, remove plaque with two to three movements of the floss toward the contact. Move floss over (C) the papilla and repeat on the adjacent tooth.

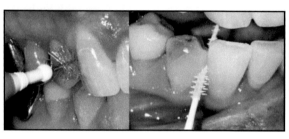

Figure 5-17. Interdental brushes: Effective devices to use for cleaning between teeth where the space below contacts allow. A variety of sizes and configurations are available. The appropriate size and shape should be selected, and interdental brushes should not be forced into spaces where they do not fit.

- Water-jet devices
  - More costly and less portable
  - Can deliver therapeutic mouth rinses
  - Multiple sizes and configurations of tips available

Dental floss (recommended for patients with good periodontal health and adequate manual dexterity) should be used as follows:

- Secure the floss around fingers on each hand or with devices so that it can be controlled and held taut.
- Gently work it through the contact between the two teeth. Some contacts are very tight, and some are not actually in contact.
- Curve the floss around one of the two teeth with fingers approximately 0.5-inch apart, and gently slide the floss into the sulcus (Figure 5-16). Pull it tightly against the tooth and move it toward the contact (the biting surface). Repeat two to three times.
- Lift the floss over the interdental papilla (the triangle of gingiva that fills the space below the contact) without the necessity of going through the contact. Curve around the adjacent tooth, and clean that surface, keeping in mind that the goal is to remove plaque from the surfaces of the teeth, not to remove debris from between the teeth.
- Lift the floss out through the contact and move to the next contact area; repeat until all interdental spaces are cleaned.

Interdental brushes (recommended where space below the contact allows their insertion) should be used as follows:

- Select a brush of the correct size for the interdental spaces to be cleaned.
- Gently slide the brush between the teeth on the gingival side of the contact (Figure 5-17).

- Using a scrubbing motion, first clean one tooth and then the other, keeping in mind that the goal is to remove plaque from the surfaces of the teeth, not to remove debris from between the teeth.
- Remove the brush and move to the next interdental space until all have been cleaned.
- The caries preventive benefit of interdental cleaning will be enhanced by applying a fluoride-containing product with the brush.

Water-jet cleaners should be used as follows:

- Use before brushing to ensure retention of the fluoride from the use of toothpaste when brushing.
- Specific instructions are provided by the manufacturers, but the key elements are as follows:
  - Select an appropriate tip.
  - Fill the reservoir with warm water or, if preferred, a mixture of mouth rinse and water (no more than 1:1 per manufacturer recommendation).
  - With the tip in the sink, prime the line to bring fluid to the tip.
  - Starting at the back of the mouth, place the tip at the gingival margin pointing toward the tooth.
  - Bend over the sink and turn on the unit with the mouth open wide enough to allow the water to flow into the sink but closed enough to avoid splashing countertops and mirrors.
  - Keeping the tip at the gingival margin, slowly move along each tooth, pausing at each interdental space to allow adequate cleansing.
  - Continue until all surfaces have been cleaned.

PREVENTIVE MANAGEMENT OF HIGH/EXTREME CARIES RISK

Persons with hyposalivation are, by definition, at high or extreme risk for caries, and, as with the case presented at the beginning of this chapter, their disease is challenging to manage, requiring multiple adjunctive interventions. In an extensive review of the literature, Gluzman, Katz, Frey, and McGowan (2013) listed four agents (sodium or stannous fluoride, chlorhexidine gluconate [CHX], amorphous calcium phosphate, and silver diamine fluoride [SDF]) that have been found to be effective in the primary prevention of root caries, alone or in combination. Because the disease process is much the same for root and coronal caries, a similar effect can be predicted for coronal caries. Other agents, such as the antimicrobial triclosan, xylitol, other polyol sugars, and the ones listed previously, have been delivered in various vehicles (i.e., dentifrice, paste, gel, varnish, lozenges, chewing gum, and mouthwashes) and should be considered as supplemental therapies. In the high-risk population of individuals with diminished salivary flow, a most aggressive approach using all available strategies must be taken to control oral diseases, especially dental caries.

Fluoride

The first line of defense in caries prevention is the use of fluoride to reduce rates of demineralization and enhance remineralization. The conversion of hydroxyapatite to fluorapatite results in enamel and dentin with lower solubility. Acid on the surface of the tooth increases porosity, enhancing the uptake of fluoride (Mount et al., 2016). Fluoride is available in many forms, and its efficacy is influenced by the concentration, volume (Paiva et al., 2017), frequency, and duration of contact with the tooth structure. Fluoridated water consumed during tooth development results in higher amounts of fluorapatite in the entire tooth and provides a continuous reservoir of low-concentration fluoride ions to contribute to remineralization. Over-the-counter (OTC) fluoride dentifrices (i.e., sodium fluoride, stannous fluoride, and sodium monofluorophosphate) with a concentration of 900 to 1500 ppm fluoride ions are recognized as effective anticaries agents

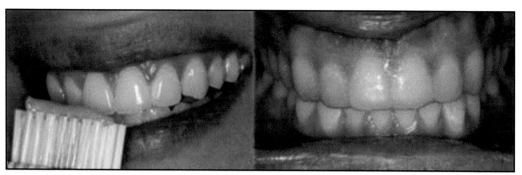

Figure 5-18. The application of caries prevention/remineralizing agents by brush or in a tray. The body of evidence supports the use of 1.1% neutral sodium fluoride once or twice daily for adolescents and adults at high risk for caries.

(Zero, 2006). Although they are regulated by the U.S. Food and Drug Administration (FDA) as OTC drugs, their formulations have changed over time without continuing evaluation of efficacy. Sodium fluoride–containing mouth rinses, available in 0.02% and 0.05% concentrations, have been found to be effective in caries reduction and may lead to higher oral fluoride retention, providing a reservoir for a greater period of time (Zero, 2006). Higher-concentration fluoride products (1.1% NaF/5000 ppm F) have been demonstrated to reduce enamel and root caries (Srinivasan, Kavitha & Loganathan, 2010; Srinivasan et al., 2014) and arrest disease progression. The products require a prescription in the United States and are available as a gel for administration in trays or as a dentifrice for brushing (Figure 5-18). Tray application may increase the duration of contact but has the potential of reducing compliance because it is an additional step, and brushing is routine for many people. Fluoride varnish (5% NaF/22,500 ppm F) administered professionally two to four times per year inhibits demineralization and promotes remineralization of enamel and dentin. The ADA has recommended its use for children, and expert opinion recommends its use in adults to prevent caries (Carey, 2014). Pediatricians are applying fluoride varnish to the teeth of at-risk children, and its application to at-risk adults by medical care providers in addition to dental providers is recommended by the American Public Health Association (2018). The FDA has approved fluoride varnish as a safe medical device for desensitizing hypersensitive teeth. In the absence of long-term studies in the United States to confirm the findings of trials completed in other countries that show its safety and efficacy as an anticaries agent, its use in the United States is off label. SDF (38%) has been used outside the United States since the 1970s. Approved by the FDA in 2014 as a desensitizing agent, like fluoride varnish, its use as an anticaries agent is an off-label use allowed by the ADA with a billing code as an interim caries arresting agent (Hendre, Taylor, Chavez, & Hyde, 2017). The fluoride content of SDF remineralizes and inhibits demineralization in enamel as with other fluoride products, but the silver has the added benefit of acting on the carious dentin to arrest the disease process. In a systematic review, Hendre et al. (2017) identified three clinical trials that support the use of SDF for the prevention and arrest of root caries with older adults. Most studies on the efficacy of SDF on the prevention of coronal caries were conducted on children, but the efficacy of the agent suggests the likelihood of equal efficacy in caries prevention in adults.

Management Strategies

The CAMBRA philosophy builds on the risk established by their CRA tool to determine patient-specific preventive programs as follows (Young & Featherstone, 2013):
- Low to moderate caries risk
  - An OTC dentifrice that contains fluoride with or without the addition of an OTC fluoride varnish (5%) at regular dental preventive appointments

- High to extreme caries risk (all people with xerostomia)
  ○ Sodium fluoride dentifrice (1.1%/5000 ppm) once or twice per day
  ○ Fluoride varnish (5%/22,500 ppm) every 3 to 4 months
  ○ SDF (38%)
    ▪ May replace the varnish, especially in the presence of exposed roots, pending additional research with adults
    ▪ Recommended frequency not established

Several considerations may have an impact on determining the most appropriate caries prevention strategies for individual patients. The OTC products are readily available and reasonably inexpensive but have limited efficacy as caries preventive agents in high-risk populations (i.e., those with diminished salivary flow by definition). The 5000 ppm sodium fluoride products are effective but require a prescription and are more expensive. Fluoride varnish requires professional application, increasing the cost to the patient. SDF is relatively inexpensive but does require professional application. An added disadvantage is that it stains carious dentin black. If these products and professional services can prevent the need for continuing restorative care and replacement of lost teeth, the presumption is that they would be cost-effective, but data to support the inference are not available.

Antimicrobial Agents

In an attempt to reduce disease risk by controlling biofilm development, various antimicrobial agents have been incorporated into oral care products. Because a biofilm is natural and beneficial to the host, the challenge is to deliver a measurable and clinically meaningful outcome without disrupting the normal oral flora. Elimination of the biofilm would be harmful to the host, but OTC oral products target drug-tolerant biofilms and are in the mouth for short periods of time at sublethal concentrations, with the result that they may selectively act on the microorganisms that cause caries and gingivitis (Marsh et al., 2015).

Triclosan with a copolymer to increase retention as an additive to a fluoride-containing dentifrice has been shown to reduce plaque, gingival inflammation, and coronal and root caries compared with a fluoride toothpaste without the triclosan/copolymer (Riley & Lamont, 2013). The use of a sonic toothbrush compared with a manual brush resulted in increased penetration of the triclosan into the biofilm that was protected from the mechanical action of the toothbrush bristles (Jongsma et al., 2015).

Arginine in the saliva has been correlated with caries resistance and serves as a substrate for arginolytic microorganisms to produce alkaline, neutralizing the acid in the biofilm (Agnello et al., 2017). In vitro, arginine impairs the growth of *S mutans* in biofilm, favors the growth of commensal arginolytic bacteria (He et al., 2016), and may act synergistically with fluoride to both alter the ecology of the plaque (Zheng et al., 2015) and promote the uptake of fluoride in enamel (Cheng et al., 2015). Although early research appears promising (Fontana, 2016; Xue et al., 2017), the evidence to support the recommendation to replace conventional fluoride toothpaste with products containing arginine is not strong (Ástvaldsdóttir et al., 2016) or, at a minimum, would be enhanced by independent studies (Fontana, 2016).

CHX is available in North America as a CHX-thymol varnish and a mouth rinse at 0.12%, and is available in formulations with and without alcohol. The prescription rinse is an effective broad-spectrum antimicrobial used twice daily. Unlike the OTC products previously discussed, its duration of action is enhanced by its substantivity to oral mucosa, biofilm, and tooth structure. The nature of the binding to both organic and inorganic substrates is not well understood and may represent differing mechanisms. The substantivity of CHX to dentin may be strengthened by the interaction of binding with hydroxyapatite by one mechanism and with the organic components of the dentin matrix by a different mechanism (Fontana, 2016).

CHX is well accepted as an antiplaque agent to reduce gingivitis (Newman et al., 2011), but evidence to support or reject it as an anticaries agent is inconclusive (Zhang, van Palenstein Helderman, van't Hof, & Truin, 2006). In a clinically relevant trial, adults with xerostomia demonstrated a reduction in new caries, especially root caries with 10% CHX varnish compared with a placebo (Banting et al., 2000). CHX has been shown to reduce salivary mutans streptococci as a marker for caries activity with CHX varnish (Patel et al., 2017), with gels being more effective than mouth rinses, which demonstrated no long-term effect (Ribeiro, Hashizume, & Maltz, 2007). The use of CHX mouth rinse is not recommended as an anticaries agent for persons with diminished salivary flow because it does not appear to be effective, and the alcohol base of most formulations acts as an astringent that will further dry oral tissues (Newman et al., 2011). However, its adherence to dentin, limited clinical studies, and the weight of professional opinion do support the use of CHX gel or CHX-thymol varnish as an adjunctive agent to manage root caries in high-risk populations (Figuero et al., 2017; Gluzman et al., 2013; Marsh et al., 2015). The application of 1.1% CHX-thymol every 3 months is recommended for the reduction of root caries but not for coronal caries (Rethman et al., 2011).

Xylitol/Sucrose-Free Polyol Chewing Gum and Lozenges

The polyols, or sugar alcohols, such as sorbitol and xylitol, are lower-calorie sweetening agents that do not cause sudden increases in blood glucose and do not promote dental caries (Calorie Control Council, 2017). In studies with children, the supervised use of chewing gum and lozenges that contain xylitol or other sucrose-free polyol after meals resulted in a reduction of new caries (Rethman et al., 2011), and systematic reviews have concluded that the regular use of xylitol and/or other polyol-containing gums and lozenges is an effective adjunct to a caries control program (Fontana, 2016). Some evidence suggests that a fluoride dentifrice that contains xylitol may be more effective at caries prevention than a fluoride-only dentifrice (Riley, Moore, Ahmed, Sharif, & Worthington, 2015). Xylitol has a dose-dependent direct effect on *S mutans* viability, adhesion to tooth structure, and acid production (Nayak, Nayak, & Khandelwal, 2014). Whether the caries preventive benefit is caused directly by xylitol on *S mutans* or indirectly by increasing the flow of saliva to dilute, buffer, and remove cariogenic microorganisms, acids, and sugars, the frequent use of these products is a recommended adjunct to a caries control program and is discussed further in the section on salivary stimulation.

Casein Phosphopeptide–Amorphous Calcium Phosphate

A variety of casein-derived calcium-based strategies have been proposed as an addition or alternative to fluoride to remineralize tooth structure. The most commonly used products contain casein phosphopeptide–amorphous calcium phosphate (CPP-ACP) or casein phosphopeptide–amorphous calcium fluoride phosphate. The proposed mechanism is that the CPP-ACP enters the porosities created by the lesion and diffuses into the lesion, providing calcium and phosphate ions to remineralize the lesion. Although fluoride remineralizes the surface of the tooth structure, the casein-derived products infiltrate deeper into the demineralized enamel. Although several reviews have concluded that these products are promising for short-term remineralization, caries prevention (Yengopal & Mickenautsch, 2009), and reducing the appearance of white spot lesions associated with orthodontic treatment (Hani, O'Connell, & Duane, 2016), fluoride remains the intervention with the most evidence to support its role in both caries prevention and the remineralization of early lesions (Memarpour, Fakhraei, Dadaein, & Vossoughi, 2015). More research is required to state definitively that the casein-derived products do have a clinically significant role in caries control in the high-risk population of those with hyposalivation (Fontana, 2016) and, if so, to determine whether it is synergistic (Srinivasan et al., 2014) with fluoride or an alternative (Oliveira et al., 2014). As a derivative of milk, CPP-ACP has been proposed as a caries-preventive food additive (Reynolds, 1998). These products do not contain lactose but should not be used by people who are allergic to milk (GC America Inc., 2018).

Diet

Although the importance of effective plaque control and the use of adjunctive agents must be part of the disease control regimen for all people, particularly for those at high risk, the most significant contributor to dental caries is diet (Moynihan & Kelly, 2014). The presence of fermentable carbohydrates is essential for shifting the ecologic balance toward an acidic biofilm that demineralizes tooth structure, leading to dental caries and/or erosion/corrosion. Sucrose provides the substrate that promotes adhesion to *S mutans* and related organisms, establishing a biofilm that selects for their survival and reproduction and becomes more cariogenic. The elimination of sucrose from the diet will control and probably completely eliminate caries (Newman et al., 2011). Accomplishing a sucrose-free diet requires not just the elimination of recognized sweets but also the elimination of most processed foods that very often contain sucrose. In an attempt to reduce dietary sugar, consumers must learn to read labels to recognize the sugar content of products and need to recognize words such as cane syrup that are used in lieu of the word "sugar." To satisfy the desire for sweet foods, several types of artificial sweeteners are available. They provide some degree of satisfaction but are often placed into highly acidic beverages that may result in dental erosion/corrosion. The alcohol sugars (polyols) used in many products do not support the growth of *S mutans,* and are thus not cariogenic, but they do have the potential side effects of bowel gas and diarrhea. Because many of the medications that cause altered salivary flow also cause constipation, some people may find the side effect a benefit. High-fructose corn syrup (HFCS) is used extensively by the food industry as a replacement for sucrose. In an in vitro study, *S mutans* grown in HFCS did not develop the robust adherence ability as that grown in sucrose, but the HFCS *S mutans* was more acidogenic (Ma et al., 2013), suggesting that HFCS cannot be recommended as a substitute for sucrose in a caries risk population. The World Health Organization strongly recommends the reduction of intake of free sugars to less than 10% of the total caloric intake and further suggests the reduction to less than 5% based on limited dose–response relationships between free sugars and caries experience (World Health Organization, 2015; Moynihan & Kelly, 2014). The U.S. diet derives approximately 13% of its energy from sugar. For control of caries, reduction of both the amount of sucrose and other fermentable carbohydrates in the diet and the frequency of their intake and duration in the mouth are essential. For individuals at high risk, it is critical. Because the diets of people with xerostomia are already influenced by difficulty with dry, salty, and spicy foods, health care professionals must coordinate to customize dietary recommendations that are both satisfying to the individual and health promoting.

Salivary Stimulation and Salivary Replacement

The best strategy for hyposalivation is to stimulate the production of saliva. In the presence of salivary glands that are not functional due to disease, radiation, and medications, the best strategy is not a viable one, but every avenue to maximize the production of saliva should be used. Pharmacological agents, such as pilocarpine and cevimeline, to stimulate salivation are covered extensively in Chapter 8. The use of gum and candies sweetened with polyols stimulates salivary flow to provide the biologically critical components to build a healthy biofilm, and may have the added benefit of the direct action of the alcohol sugars on *S mutans.* The gum and/or candies should be used frequently throughout the day for maximum benefit. One interesting product is a bilayer lozenge that contains xylitol and has a vegetable gum adhesive on one side. One to two lozenges are

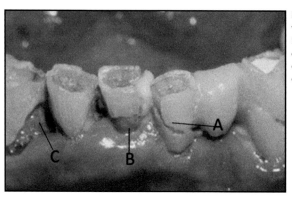

Figure 5-19. The patient was previously treated with head and neck radiation for pharyngeal cancer. He carried a cup containing cola that he sipped constantly to ease the discomfort of his extremely dry mouth. He presented with (A) eroded/corroded enamel, (B) demineralized dentin, and (C) root caries.

placed on the gingiva or oral mucosa, and the xylitol is slowly released; the time varies from person to person but averages 1.18 hours. Participants reported a perceived increase in oral wetness upon waking and decreased oral discomfort (Burgess & Lee, 20121). The selection of products will be based on patient preference, but care should be advised to avoid highly acidic products that may result in erosion (University of Florida, 2018). Intense mint or cinnamon flavorings may be an irritant to oral mucosa that lacks the protective layer that saliva provides.

With an aging population and the medications associated with age-related diseases, an increasing number of products are being marketed for alleviating the symptoms of dry mouth. Saliva substitutes in various formulations are available (e.g., sprays, gels, pastes, swabs, rinses). Formulations vary, but most contain carboxymethylcellulose or glycerin to act as a lubricant, water, xylitol or other polyols, and flavoring agents. Salivary substitutes have little therapeutic value but may make a significant contribution to quality of life for some individuals. Depending on the constituents of the product, they may also serve as a vehicle for the delivery of sufficient polyols to alter *S mutans* or fluoride to remineralize the tooth structure. The lubricating effect is transient and may provide a short-term benefit in easing speech and swallowing. Many people become accustomed to the oral dryness and find it difficult to adapt to the change to an unfamiliar lubricated mucosa. To assist people in determining if the products will improve comfort, it may be useful to recommend that the products be used on a scheduled basis for a trial period (e.g., every 2 hours during waking hours for 2 to 4 weeks). The selection of products should be based on patient preference (i.e., taste, texture, and convenience). From a professional perspective, one major concern is the acidity of certain products that may further increase the potential of erosion and contribute to tipping the ecological balance of the biofilm to becoming more cariogenic in this high-risk population. Professional recommendations should be for products that have a pH of 6.7 or higher and preferably contain fluoride and calcium (Delgado & Olafsson, 2017; University of Florida, 2018).

An obvious and often overlooked way to provide oral moisture and ensure adequate hydration is frequent sipping of water. Simply carrying water bottles or covered cups with water or ice affords the availability of access at any time. Education is essential to ensure that people understand that the fluid must be water and not a sweetened or acidic beverage. A veteran patient who had been treated with radiation for pharyngeal cancer was referred to the Veterans Affairs dental clinic. He entered the clinic carrying his cup and reported that this was his usual practice. However, his cup contained cola. Much of his enamel had dissolved due to erosion/corrosion, and the exposed dentin was so thoroughly demineralized that it had a rubbery consistency, resulting in teeth that were at risk of fracturing off completely and were essentially unrestorable (Figure 5-19).

Professional Dental Care

The recommendation that people see their dentist twice per year may have had its origin from an Ipana toothpaste ad from the 1950s and has become somewhat institutionalized in dentistry and by the dental insurance industry (Stefanac, Nesbit, & Armfield, 2017). Systematic reviews have found little evidence to support or refute the practice of semiannual preventive care (Riley, Worthington, Clarkson, & Bierne, 2013), but expert opinion unequivocally states that intervals between routine appointments must be patient specific. The ADA published "that the frequency of [patients'] regular dental visits should be tailored by their dentists to accommodate for their current oral health status and health history. Based on data analysis, researchers speculate that high-risk patients would likely benefit from more frequent dental visits, while low-risk patients may see the same benefits from only one cleaning per year" (ADA, 2013). Patients at high risk for caries and patients with hyposalivation are by definition at high or extreme caries risk; patients with periodontitis must be on an aggressive maintenance program and should be seen by a dental professional at least every 3 months. Procedures to be done at the periodic preventive appointments, recall, or recare visits (interchangeable terms in dentistry) must be tailored to the health needs of the patient. For the patient with xerostomia, the dentition and oral tissues should be thoroughly examined because disease, especially dental caries, can progress extremely rapidly in the absence of the protection of saliva. Skills at disrupting plaque should be assessed and individualized education provided to ensure the patient is able to effectively brush and achieve interdental cleaning. The dentist or dental hygienist should apply fluoride varnish or SDF and be certain that the patient has an adequate supply or current prescription for 5000 ppm fluoride. Everyone who interacts with the patient should emphasize the importance of maintaining a sugar intake that is low in both amount and frequency. Referral for dental consultation must be part of the comprehensive management of patients with hyposalivation.

Dentures

Teeth that have been lost due to caries, periodontal disease, or trauma are replaced in multiple ways, such as implants and full or partial dentures. Each has its own challenges for maintaining health. Implant restorations require meticulous control of plaque biofilm to prevent loss due to peri-implantitis, a risk probably enhanced by xerostomia. In people with removable full or partial dentures, saliva acts as a lubricant to allow the prosthesis (denture) to move against the mucosa while chewing and speaking without being abrasive, and it provides an interface that creates adhesion between the denture and the tissue. In the absence of adequate salivary flow, denture (pressure) ulcers and mucosal irritation are common, and retention of dentures is reduced. The use of salivary replacement gels placed on the contact surface of the prosthesis may be particularly helpful for both retention and comfort, but wearers of dentures with dry mouths may have to rely on denture adhesives. Dentures cover mucosal tissues, providing a rich breeding ground for the growth of bacteria and fungi (*C albicans*). In a mouth with normal salivary function, it is important to have the dentures out of the mouth for some period of each day and to keep them cleaned to protect the tissues that they contact. For those without the protection of saliva, denture cleanliness is essential, and tissues must have some time free of the prosthesis.

THE FUTURE

Successful treatment of xerostomia and salivary hypofunction is of interest to both patients and researchers. Gaps in our understanding of Sjögren's syndrome and head-and-neck radiation need to be bridged for the development of effective treatments. Ongoing breakthroughs in gene therapy, stem cell therapy, and tissue engineering show great promise for future therapies. (Quock, 2016, p. 57)

Knowledge gaps about oral disease pathogenesis and prevention require continuing exploration with the development of solutions that might establish a beneficial biofilm or more effectively remineralize the tooth structure when compromised salivary function creates an environment that predisposes to disease. In the interim, people with diminished salivation require comprehensive interdisciplinary care and a health care system that provides access to needed services and therapies. Ideally, care might be provided by a team of care providers who understand the complexities of xerostomia and share the plans of care. An essential first step is for all potential members of the team to understand what all the others provide and how their roles might be expanded to improve patient comfort and reduce disease risk. Medical care providers might consider applying fluoride varnish or prescribing 1.1% neutral sodium fluoride. Nutritionists can develop a diet that has low cariogenicity and is accepted by the individual. Pharmacists could provide recommendations that might reduce drug side effects and improve salivary function. Dental personnel might identify patients who need medical or dietary interventions. At the core, effective mechanisms for interdisciplinary communication and referral are essential.

REFERENCES

Agnello, M., Cen, L., Tran, N. C., Shi, W., McLean, J. S., & He, X. (2017). Arginine improves pH homeostasis via metabolism and microbiome modulation. *Journal of Dental Research, 96*(8), 924-930. doi:10.1177/0022034517707512

Akpan, A., & Morgan, R. (2002). Oral candidiasis. *Postgraduate Medical Journal, 78*(922), 455-459. doi:10.1136/pmj.78.922.455

American Dental Association (2011). Caries risk assessment form. Retrieved from http://www.ada.org/~/media/ADA/Science%20and%20Research/Files/topic_caries_over6.ashx

American Dental Association. (2013). *American Dental Association Statement on Regular Dental Visits.* Retrieved from https://www.ada.org/en/press-room/news-releases/2013-archive/june/american-dental-association-statement-on-regular-dental-visits

American Dental Association. (2018). You can prevent tooth decay by following these tips. Retrieved from https://www.mouthhealthy.org/en/az-topics/d/decay

American Public Health Association. (2018). Evidence-based dental care. Retrieved from https://www.apha.org/policies-and-advocacy/public-health-policy-statements/policy-database/2014/07/09/13/29/evidence-based-dental-care

Arweiler, N. B., & Netuschil, L. (2016). The oral microbiota. *Advances in Experimental Medicine and Biology, 902,* 45-60.

Ástvaldsdóttir, Á., Naimi-Akbar, A., Davidson, T., Brolund, A., Lintamo, L., Attergren Granath, A., … Östlund, P. (2016). Arginine and caries prevention: A systematic review. *Caries Research, 50,* 383-393. doi:10.1159/000446249

Banting, D. W., Papas, A., Clark, D. C., Proskin, H. M., Schultz, M., & Perry, R. (2000). The effectiveness of 10% chlorhexidine varnish treatment on dental caries incidence in adults with dry mouth. *Gerodontology, 17*(2), 67-76. doi:10.1111/j.1741-2358.2000. 00067.x

Bass, C. C. (1954). An effective method of personal oral hygiene; Part II. *Journal of the Louisiana State Medical Society, 106,* 110-112.

Billings, M., Dye, B., Iafolla, T., Grisius, M., & Alevizos, I. (2017). Elucidating the role of hyposalivation and autoimmunity in oral candidiasis. *Oral Diseases, 23*(3), 387-394. doi:10.111/odi.12626

Burgess, J., & Lee, P. (2011). XyliMelts time-release adhering discs for night-time oral dryness. *International Journal of Dental Hygiene, 10*(2), 118-121. doi:10.111/j.1601-5037.2011.00532.x

Buzalaf, M., Hannas, A., & Kato, M. (2012). Saliva and dental erosion. *Journal of Applied Oral Science, 20*(5), 493-502. doi:10.1590/s1678-77572012000500001

Calorie Control Council. (2017). Facts about polyols: Polyols and gastrointestinal (GI) effects. Retrieved from https://polyols.org/frequently-asked-questions/fap-g

Carey, C. M. (2014). Focus on fluorides: Update on the use of fluoride for the prevention of dental caries. *Journal of Evidence-Based Dental Practice, 14*, 95-102. doi:10.1016/j.jebdp.2014.02.004

Chapple, I. L., Van der Weijden, F., Doerfer, C., Herrera, D., Shapira, L., Polak, D., … Graziani, F. (2015). Primary prevention of periodontitis: Managing gingivitis. *Journal of Clinical Periodontology, 42*(Suppl. 16), S71-S76. doi:10.111/jcpe.12366

Cheng, X., Xu, P., Zhou, X., Deng, M., Cheng, M., Li, M., … Xu, X. (2015). Arginine promotes fluoride uptake into artificial carious lesions in vitro. *Australian Dental Journal, 60*(1), 104-111. doi:10.111/adj.12278

Dawes, C., Pedersen, A. M., Villa, A., Ekstrom, J., Proctor, G. B., Vissink, A., … Wolff, A. (2015). The functions of human saliva: A review sponsored by the World Workshop on Oral Medicine VI. *Archives of Oral Biology 60*(6), 863-874. doi:10.1016/j.archoralbio.2015.03.004

Delgado, A. J., & Olafsson, V. G. (2017). Acidic oral moisturizers with pH below 6.7 may be harmful to teeth depending on formulation: A short report. *Clinical, Cosmetic and Investigational Dentistry, 9*, 81-83. doi:10.2147/CCIDE.S140254

Donlan, R. M. (2002). Biofilms: Microbial life on surfaces. *Emerging Infectious Diseases, 8*(9), 881-890. doi:103201/eid0809.020063

Dye, B. A., Thornton-Evans, G., Li, X., & Iafolla, T. (2015). *Dental caries and tooth loss in adults in the United States, 2011-2012.* Hyattsville, MD: U.S. Department of Health and Human Services, Centers for Disease Control and Prevention, National Center for Health Statistics.

Featherstone, J. (2008). Dental caries: A dynamic disease process. *Australian Dental Journal, 53*(3), 286-291. doi:10.1111/j.1834-7819.2008.00064.x

Featherstone, J. D., & Chaffee, B. W. (2018) The Evidence for Caries Management by Risk Assessment (CAMBRA®). *Advances in Dental Research, 29*(1), 9-14.

Featherstone, J. D., White, J. M., Hoover, C. I., Rapozo-Hilo, M., Weintraub, J. A., Zhan, L., Gansky, S. A. (2012). A randomized clinical trial of anticaries therapies targeted according to risk assessment (caries management by risk assessment). *Caries Res, 2012;46*(2):118-129.

Figuero, E., Nobrega, D. F., Garcia-Gargallo, M., Tenuta, L M., Herrera, D., & Carvalho, J. C. (2017). Mechanical and chemical plaque control in the simultaneous management of gingivitis and caries: A systematic review. *Journal of Clinical Periodontology, 44*(S18), S116-S134. doi:10.1111/jcpe.12674

Fontana, M. (2016). Enhancing fluoride: Clinical human studies of alternatives or boosters for caries management. *Caries Research, 50*(1), 22-37. doi:10.1159/000439059

Friedman, P. K. (2014). *Geriatric dentistry: Caring for our aging population.* Ames, IA: Wiley Blackwell.

Gao, X., Jiang, S., Koh, D., & Hsu, C. S. (2016). Salivary biomarkers for dental caries. *Periodontology 2000, 70*(1), 128-141. doi:10.1111/prd.12100

GC America Inc. (2018). MI Paste family microsite—Frequently asked questions (FAQs). Retrieved from http://www.mi-paste.com/FAQ/F.php

Gluzman, R., Katz, R. V., Frey, B. J., & McGowan, R. (2013). Prevention of root caries: A literature review of primary and secondary preventive agents. *Special Care in Dentistry, 33*(3), 133-140. doi:10.1111/j.1754-4505.2012.00318.x

Hani, T. B., O'Connell, A., & Duane, B. (2016). Casein phosphopeptide–amorphous calcium phosphate products in caries prevention. *Evidence-Based Dentistry 17*, 46-47. doi:10.1038/sf.ebd.6401168

Hannig, C., Hannig, M., Kensche, A., & Carpenter, G. (2017). The mucosal pellicle–An underestimated factor in oral physiology. *Archives of Oral Biology, 80*, 144-152. doi:10.1016/j.archoralbio.2017.04.001

He, J., Hwang, G., Liu, Y., Gao, L., Kilpatrick-Liverman, L., Santarpia, P., … Koo, H. (2016). L-arginine modifies the exopolysaccharide matrix and thwarts Streptococcus mutans outgrowth within mixed-species oral biofilms. *Journal of Bacteriology, 198*(19), 2651-61. doi:10.1128/JB.00021-16

Hendre, A. D., Taylor, G. W., Chavez, E. M., & Hyde, S. (2017). A systematic review of silver diamine fluoride: Effectiveness and application in older adults. *Gerodontology, 34*(4), 411-419. doi:10.1111/ger.12294

Holm-Pedersen, P., Walls, A. W., & Ship, J. A. (2015) *Textbook of geriatric dentistry.* Chichester, United Kingdom: John Wiley & Sons.

Jain, S., & Jain, H. (2017). Legendary hero: Dr. G.V. Black (1836-1915). *Journal of Clinical and Diagnostic Research, 11*(5), ZB01-ZB04.

Jepsen, S., Blanco, J., Buchalla, W., Carvalho, J. C., Dietrich, T., Dorfer, C., … Machiulsience, V. (2017). Prevention and control of dental caries and periodontal diseases at individual and population level: Consensus report of group 3 of joint EFP/ORCA workshop on the boundaries between caries and periodontal diseases. *Journal of Clinical Periodontology, 44*(S18), S85-S93. doi:10.1111/jcpe.12687

Jongsma, M. A., van de Lagemaat, M., Busscher, H. J., Geertzema-Doornbusch, G. I., Alema-Smit, J., van der Mei, H. C., & Ren, Y. (2015). Synergy of brushing mode and antibacterial use on in vivo biofilm formation. *Journal of Dentistry, 43*(12), 1580-1586. doi:10.1016/j.jdent.2015.08.001

Kaidonis, J., & Townsend, G. (2016). The 'sialo–microbial–dental complex' in oral health and disease. *Annals of Anatomy, 203*, 85-89. doi:10.1016/j.s0940-9602(13)00010-1

Kanzow, P., Wegehaupt, F. J., Attin, T., & Wiegand, A. (2016). Etiology and pathogenesis of dental erosion. *Quintessence International, 47*(4), 275-278.

Kassenbaum, N. J., Smith, A. G. C., Bernabe, E., Fleming, T. D., Reynolds, A. E., Vos, T., ... Marcenes, W. (2017). Global, regional, and national prevalence, incidence, and disability—Adjusted life years for oral conditions for 195 countries, 1990-2015: A systematic analysis for the global burden of diseases, injuries, and risk factors. *Journal of Dental Research, 96*(4):380-387. doi:10.1177/0022034517693566

Kilian, M., Chapple, I. L., Hannig, M., Marsh, P. D., Meuric, V., Pedersen, A. M., ... Zaura, E. (2016). The oral microbiome—An update for oral healthcare professionals. *British Dental Journal, 221*(10), 657-666. doi:10.1038/sj.bdj.2016.865

Kotsakis, G. A., Lian, Q., Ioannou, A. L., Michalowicz, B. S., John, M. T., & Chu, H. (2018). A network meta-analysis of interproximal oral hygiene methods in the reduction of clinical indices of inflammation. *Journal of Periodontology, 89*(5), 558-570. doi:10.1002/jper.17-0368

Kumar, S., Tadakamadia, J., & Johnson, N. W. (2016). Effect of toothbrushing frequency on incidence and increment of dental caries: A systematic review and meta-analysis. *Journal of Dental Research, 95*(11), 1230-1236.

Lendenmann, U., Grogan, J., & Oppenheim, F. (2000). Saliva and dental pellicle—A review. *Advances in Dental Research, 14*(1), 22-28. doi:10.1177/08959374000140010301

Lertpimonchai, A., Rattanasiri, S., Arj-Ong Vallibhakara, S., Attia, J., & Thakkinstian, A. (2017). The association between oral hygiene and periodontitis: A systematic review and meta-analysis. *International Dental Journal, 67*(6), 332-343. doi:10.1111/idj.12317

Marchesan, J., Morelli, T., Moss, K., Preisser, J., Zandona, A., Offenbacher, S., & Beck, J. (2018). Interdental cleaning is associated with decreased oral disease prevalence. *Journal of Dental Research, 97*(7), 773-778. doi:10.1177/0022034518759915

Marsh, P. D., Head, D. A., & Devine, D. A. (2015). Ecological approaches to oral biofilms: Control without killing. *Caries Research, 49*(1), 46-54. doi:10.1159/000377732

Memarpour, M., Fakhraei, E., Dadaein, S., & Vossoughi, M. (2015). Efficacy of fluoride varnish and casein phosphopeptide-amorphous calcium phosphate for remineralization of primary teeth: A randomized clinical trial. *Medical Principles and Practice, 24*(3), 231-237. doi:10.1159/000379750

Mount, G. J., Hume, W. R., Ngo, H. C., & Wolff, M. S. (2016). *Preservation and restoration of tooth structure.* Chichester, United Kingdom: John Wiley & Sons.

Moynihan, P. J., & Kelly, S. A. M. (2014). Effect on caries of restricting sugars intake: Systematic review to inform WHO guidelines. *Journal of Dental Research, 93*(1), 8-18. doi:10.1177/0022034513508954

Nayak, P. A., Nayak, U. A., & Khandelwal, V. (2014). The effect of xylitol on dental caries and oral flora. *Clinical, Cosmetic and Investigational Dentistry, 6,* 89-94. doi:10.2147/CCIDE.S55761

Newman, M. G., Takei, H. H., Klokkevold, P. R., & Carranza, F. A. (2011). *Carranza's clinical periodontology* (11th ed.). St. Louis, MO: Saunders/Elsevier.

Oliveira, G. M., Ritter, A. V., Heymann, H. Q., Swift, E., Donovan, T., Brock, G., & Wright, T. (2014). Remineralization effect of CPP-ACP and fluoride for white spot lesions in vitro. *Journal of Dentistry, 42*(12), 1592-1602. doi:101016/j.jdent.2014.09.004

Paiva, M. F., Delbem, A. C. B., Danelon, M., Nagata, M. E., Moraes, F. R. N., Coclete, G. E. G., ... Pessan, J. P. (2017). Fluoride concentration and amount of dentifrice influence enamel demineralization in situ. *Journal of Dentistry, 66,* 18-22. doi:10.1016/j.jdent.2017.09.004

Patel, P. M., Hugar, S. M., Halikerimath, S., Badakar, C. M., Gokhale, N. S., Thakkar, P. J., ... Shah. S. (2017). Comparison of the effect of fluoride varnish, chlorhexidine varnish and casein phosphopeptide-amorphous calcium phosphate (CPP-ACP) varnish on salivary streptococcus mutans level: A six-month clinical study. *Journal of Clinical and Diagnostic Research, 11*(8), ZC53-ZC59. doi:10.7860/jcdr/2017/26541.10409

Pitts, N. B., Zero, D. T., Marsh, P. D., Ekstrand, K., Weintraub, J. A., Ramos-Gomez, F., ... Ismail, A. (2017). Dental caries. *Nature Reviews Disease Primers, 3,* 17030. doi:10.1038/nrdp.2017.30

Quock, R. (2016). Xerostomia: Current streams of investigation. *Oral Surgery, Oral Medicine, Oral Pathology, and Oral Radiology, 122*(1), 53-60. doi:10.1016/j.0000.2016.03.002

Rethman, M. P., Beltran-Aguilar, E. D., Billings, R. J., Hujoel, P. P., Katz, B. P., Milgrom, P., ... Meyer, D. M. (2011). Nonfluoride caries-preventive agents: Executive summary of evidence-based clinical recommendations. *Journal of the American Dental Association 142*(9), 1065-1071.

Reynolds, E. C. (1998). Anticariogenic complexes of amorphous calcium phosphate stabilized by casein phosphopeptides: A review. *Special Care in Dentistry, 18*(1), 8-16. doi:10.1111/j.1754-4505.1998.tb01353.x

Ribeiro, L. G., Hashizume, L. N., & Maltz, M. (2007). The effect of different formulations of chlorhexidine in reducing levels of mutans streptococci in the oral cavity: A systematic review of the literature. *Journal of Dentistry 35*(5), 359-370. doi:10.1016/j.jdent.2007.01.007

Riley P., & Lamont, T. (2013). Triclosan/copolymer containing toothpastes for oral health. *Cochrane Database of Systematic Reviews, 12,* CD010514. doi:10.1002/14651858.cd010514

Riley, P., Moore, D., Ahmed, F., Sharif, M., & Worthington, H. (2015). Xylitol-containing products for preventing dental caries in children and adults. *Cochrane Database of Systematic Reviews, 36*(3), CD010743. doi:10.1002/14651858.cd010743.pub2

Riley, P., Worthington, H., Clarkson, J., & Beirne, P. (2013). Recall intervals for oral health in primary care patients. *Cochrane Database of Systematic Reviews,12*(2), CD004346. doi:10.1002/14651858.cd004346.pub4

Srinivasan, N., Kavitha, M., & Loganathan, S. (2010). Comparison of the remineralization potential of CPP-ACP and CPP-ACP with 900 ppm fluoride on eroded human enamel: An in situ study. *Archives of Oral Biology* 55(7), 541-544. doi:10.1016/j.archoralbio.2010.05.002

Srinivasan, M., Schimmel, M., Riesen, M., Ilgner, A., Wicht, M. J., Warncke, M., ... Noack, M. J. (2014). High-fluoride toothpaste: A multicenter randomized controlled trial in adults. *Community Dentistry and Oral Epidemiology, 42,* (4), 333-340. doi:10.111/cdoe.12090

Stefanac, S., Nesbit, S., & Armfield, J. (2017). *Diagnosis and treatment planning in dentistry.* St. Louis, MO: Elsevier.

University of Florida. (2018). Potential erosive assessment of dry mouth lozenges and tablets on dentin. Retrieved from https://oralacidityawareness.files.wordpress.com/2018/09/delgado_aadr_2018_acidity_of_dry_mouth_lozenges.pdf

Valkenburg, C., Slot, D. E., Bakker, E. W., & Van der Weijden, F. A. (2016). Does dentifrice use help to remove plaque? A systematic review. *Journal of Clinical Periodontology* 43(12), 1050-1058. doi:10.1111/jcpe.12615

Van der Weijden, F. A., & Slot, D. E. (2015). Efficacy of homecare regimens for mechanical plaque removal in managing gingivitis a meta review. *Journal of Clinical Periodontology, 42*(S16), S77-S91. doi:10.1111/jcpe.12359

Walton, R. E., Torabinejad, M., & Fouad, A. F. (2015). *Endodontics: Principles and practice* (5th ed.). St. Louis, MO: Elsevier/Saunders

Wheeler, R. C., & Ash, M. M. K. (1984). *Wheeler's dental anatomy, physiology, and occlusion.* Philadelphia, PA: Saunders.

World Health Organization. (2015). Guideline: Sugars intake for adults and children. Retrieved from https://apps.who.int/iris/bitstream/handle/10665/149782/9789241549028_eng.pdf;jsessionid=04253EB1614A25CDA3404A0EEB8CA85B?sequence=1

Xue, Y., Lu, Q., Tian, Y., Zhou, X., Cheng, L., & Ren, B. (2017). Effect of toothpaste containing arginine on dental plaque—A randomized controlled in situ study. *Journal of Dentistry, 67,* 88-93. doi:10.1016/j.jdent.2017.10.001

Yaacob, M., Worthington, H., Deacon, S., Deery, C., Walmsley, A., Robinson, P., & Glenny, A. (2014). Powered versus manual toothbrushing for oral health. *Cochrane Database of Systematic Reviews, 6*(6), CD002281. doi:10.1002/14651858.cd002281.pub3

Yengopal, V., & Mickenautsch, S. (2009). Caries preventive effect of casein phosphopeptide-amorphous calcium phosphate (CPP-ACP): A meta-analysis. *Acta Odontologica Scandinavica, 67*(6), 321-332. doi:10.1080/00016350903160563

Young, D. A., & Featherstone, J. D. (2013). Caries management by risk assessment. *Community Dentistry and Oral Epidemiology, 41*(1), e53-63. doi:10.1111/cdoe.12031

Young, D. A., Novy, B. B., Zeller, G. G., Hale, R. Hart, T. C., & Truelove, E. L. (2015). The American Dental Association Caries Classification System for clinical practice: A report of the American Dental Association Council on Scientific Affairs. *The Journal of the American Dental Association, 146*(2), 79-86.

Zero, D. T. (2006). Dentifrices, mouthwashes, and remineralization/caries arrestment strategies. *BMC Oral Health, 6*(Suppl. 1), S9. doi:10.1186/1472-6831-6-S1-S9

Zhang, Q., van Palenstein Helderman, W. H., van't Hof, M. A., & Truin, G. J. (2006). Chlorhexidine varnish for preventing dental caries in children, adolescents and young adults: A systematic review. *European Journal of Oral Sciences, 114*(6), 449-455. doi:10.1111/j.1600-0722.2006.00392.x

Zheng, X., Cheng, X., Wang, L., Qiu, W., Wang, S., Zhou, Y., ... Xu, X. (2015). Combinatorial effects of arginine and fluoride on oral bacteria. *Journal of Dental Research, 94*(2), 344-353. doi:10.1177/0022034514561259

6

Swallowing, Xerostomia, and Hyposalivation

Joseph Murray, PhD, CCC-SLP, BCS-S and
Rebecca H. Affoo, PhD, CCC-SLP, SLP(C), Reg. CASLPO

In this chapter, we discuss the complex relationship between the physical state of hyposalivation, the symptom of xerostomia, and the interaction between oral health and systemic health with a focused discussion related to dysphagia and aspiration pneumonia. The text includes an in-depth discussion of saliva production and components that aid in the lubrication of foods to facilitate mastication and pharyngeal transit during swallowing. Additional discussion relates the import of saliva to enable taste and as a contributor to triggering the reflexive portion of the swallow. The role of salivation in the enhancement and preservation of oral health is discussed in depth. Following this, these same topics are discussed in the context of hyposalivation and xerostomia. Each of the facilitative contributions to mastication, swallowing, and oral health is described in a way to help clinicians understand the impact of hyposalivation on the whole-body health of their patients. A review of treatments for patients with xerostomia is also provided.

Shared Pathway

Ventilation, nutrition, and hydration are compulsory for sustaining life. The oropharynx is a shared pathway that supports these functions. The transport of food and fluid through the enteral tract requires salivary secretions in order to lubricate the mouth, stimulate lower enteral secretion output, and initiate chemical digestion of starches. The preparation of the material in the oral cavity through mastication of solid food material and movement of the bolus of food or fluid from the mouth to the stomach could not be achieved without the unique properties that are inherent in salivary secretions (Miller, 2013). At rest, the shared pathway functions as an airway delivering oxygen to the relatively pristine and delicate pulmonary system from an environment that may vary between extremes of temperature and humidity and an unhealthy suspension of a multitude of microorganisms and other particulates. These threats to the body are accommodated by the constant production and clearance of secretions, which warm and humidify the air we breathe while

- 77 -

Ginsberg, S. M. (Ed.).
Xerostomia: An Interdisciplinary Approach
to Managing Dry Mouth (pp. 77-97).
© 2020 Taylor & Francis Group.

providing a complex physical and biological barrier. Salivary secretions provide further protection against mechanical, thermal, and chemical irritation. The secretions facilitate remineralization of the teeth, deliver antimicrobial actions by clearing pathogens from the oral cavity and pharynx, initiate chemical digestion, and enable taste (Whelton, 2004).

SALIVA AND ITS EFFECTS ON BOLUS PREPARATION AND SWALLOWING

Swallowing is a complex sensorimotor phenomenon and the process by which saliva, food, and fluid are transported from the mouth to the stomach (Jean, 1984; Matsuo & Jeffery, 2013), while the upper respiratory tract is simultaneously protected from pulmonary aspiration of the material being swallowed (Bosma, 1957). Alimentary swallowing is composed of an anticipatory phase consisting of manual preparation of food before inserting it into the oral cavity. This is followed by an oral preparatory phase consisting of lingual, labial, and masticatory manipulations of the food.

Mastication

The purpose of mastication is to process food in the oral cavity into a bolus that can be transported through the oropharynx, swallowed safely, and then easily digested (Pedersen, Bardow, Jensen, & Nauntofte, 2002; van der Bilt, Engelen, Pereira, van der Glas, & Abbink, 2006). During mastication, ingested food particles are mechanically reduced in size through the process of lingual particle selection and fragmentation between the occlusal surfaces of the teeth (Thexton, 1992). Factors such as the total occlusal area; number of teeth; bite force; and coordination between the movement of the jaw, tongue, and cheeks during manipulation of the food particles play an important role in effective mastication (Hiiemae, Thexton, & Crompton, 1978; Thexton, 1992; van der Bilt et al., 2006). The secretion of saliva is critical for effective mastication, bolus formation, and bolus transport, and both the volume and composition of saliva contribute significantly to these functions (Dawes et al., 2015). The water in saliva is used to moisten the food particles, allowing the salivary amylase to access available starch and initiate chemical digestion (Hoebler et al., 1998). The salivary mucins bind masticated food into a coherent and slippery bolus that can easily be transported through the oropharynx (Pedersen et al., 2002).

The secretions rich in mucins have the ability to not only lubricate but also to stretch and bond to one another to form tangled grids or webs known as *spinnbarkeit* that coat the epithelial surfaces of the mouth and pharynx. Collins and Dawes (1987) calculated that spinnbarkeit is typically present as a thin film with a depth of 70 to 100 μm. Wolff and Kleinberg (1998) reported that the film varies in thickness and is thickest on the posterior tongue and thinnest on the hard palate. When solid food is mixed with mucin-rich secretions, they serve to minimize shear stresses during mastication, allowing for less effort in masticatory cycles (Rogus-Pulia, Gangnon, Kind, Connor, & Asthana, 2018). Another study suggests that the extensional viscosity may be reduced by the shear forces in chewing and further affected by the change in pH introduced by bicarbonate in the parotid secretions (Vijay et al., 2015). It is not well understood why this change occurs, but it is likely related to the increased need to add moisture to the food being masticated and to free mucins from the spinnbarkeit to the same solid foods. During periods of rest when no chewing or swallowing occurs, saliva is secreted in a smaller volume but with a greater density of mucins, allowing for the reformation of the dense web-like tangle of mucins. During mastication, enzymes in the secretions (amylase and lipase) are ground into foods and begin the process of digestion that continues as the bolus traverses the enteral tract. These enzymes also dissolve molecules in the food that provide stimulation to the taste receptors, which in turn further stimulate the production of oropharyngeal and gastric secretions. The hardness and particle size decrease with salivary mucins, binding the masticated food into a cohesive but slippery bolus that is ready for transport through the pharynx and esophagus. The urge to swallow is triggered by a threshold level in both food particle size, when the cohesive forces between the food particles in the bolus are strongest, and lubrication of the food bolus (Hutchings & Lillford, 1988; Peyron et al., 2011; Prinz & Lucas, 1995, 1997). Thus, both masticatory performance and salivary volume and composition play an important role in preparing food to be eaten.

Taste

Saliva also contributes greatly to taste perception because it dissolves food particles and changes the molecular structure as the particles are transported to the sensory cells responsible for taste detection (Dawes et al., 2015; Running, 2018). It is known that the density of certain proteins in saliva can alter one's perception of bitter and sweet tastes. Carbonic anhydrase VI, a protein associated with bitter taste perception, is secreted from the von Ebner glands, which are minor salivary glands located near the circumvallate papillae on the tongue that have a very high density of bitter taste receptors. This arrangement suggests that there is likely an organized localization of protein production and dedicated sensory reception. This is an area of research that is only recently emerging as scientists continue to unwrap the mysteries of taste perception. Carbonic anhydrase VI has also been associated with the growth and renewal of taste buds because the levels of this protein have been observed to be reduced in individuals with abnormalities in the density of taste sensory cells (Dynesen, 2015). This protein has been suggested to sustain a healthy population of taste buds by suppressing cell apoptosis (programmed cell death) for taste sensory cells (Wang, Zhou, Brand, & Huang, 2007).

There are other proteins associated with perceptions of sweetness and fat. Subjects with higher amounts of salivary alpha-amylase were less likely to perceive the sweet sensation in foods rich in sucrose. The volume of salivary alpha-amylase has also been associated with greater food intake in obese women compared with average-weight control subjects (Harthoorn, 2008). Patients with greater levels of alpha-amylase in their saliva break down carbohydrates more rapidly. It could be further postulated that early digestion and reduced perception, along with the associated increased oral intake, may combine and synergistically lead to weight gain in those with greater levels of alpha-amylase.

The process of gustation may facilitate salivary secretion (Dietsch, Pelletier, & Solomon, 2018; Watanabe & Dawes, 1988), which may aid in forming and swallowing the bolus, supporting the view that eating is a highly interdependent process. Increased salivary secretion in response to gustation is also a protective mechanism. Noxious-tasting stimuli entering the oral cavity may be suspended in an increased volume of saliva and then expectorated from the mouth before they can potentially harm the body (Dawes et al., 2015). Gustation and subsequent salivary secretion appear to have a facilitatory effect on swallowing (Logemann et al., 1995). Sensory information related to gustation is carried through the special sensory components of the glossopharyngeal and facial cranial nerves and travels to the nucleus tractus solitarius, a sensory nuclei that is vital in triggering the pharyngeal phase of swallowing (Dodds, 1989). For a comprehensive review of the sensory input pathways and their impact on swallowing, please see Steele and Miller (2010).

Bolus Preparation

During the oral phase, the bolus is propelled posteriorly in the oral cavity toward the faucial pillars and the posterior pharyngeal tongue by a lingual stripping wave. The pharyngeal phase of the swallow is triggered, and a highly complex, stereotypical series of muscle contractions and movements occur in order for the bolus to be safely transported from the posterior oral cavity to the esophagus and down into the stomach. The role of saliva in the process of swallowing is complex and is not currently well understood. Saliva minimally provides essential lubrication within the oral cavity during the swallowing process (Hughes et al., 1987). However, recent simulation work suggests that the contribution of saliva to swallowing is more complex than merely providing oropharyngeal lubrication (Ho et al., 2017). The volume of saliva secreted into the oral cavity may influence the rate of swallowing when resting or engaging in non-alimentary activities (Kapila, Dodds, Helm, & Hogan, 1984; Nederkoorn, Smulders, & Jansen, 1999; Rudney, Ji, & Larson, 1995), and there is also evidence to suggest that the volume of saliva secreted into the oral cavity during alimentation may impact swallowing biomechanics (Rhodus, Colby, Moller, & Bereuter, 1995; Rhodus, Moller, Colby, & Bereuter, 1995; Rogus-Pulia & Logemann, 2011).

Swallowing disorders occur when deficits impact a person's ability to transport saliva, food, and fluid from the mouth to the stomach while simultaneously protecting the upper respiratory tract from pulmonary aspiration of the material being swallowed (Logemann, 1995). The major complications of dysphagia include malnutrition (Namasivayam & Steele, 2015), dehydration (Whelan, 2001), and aspiration pneumonia (Foley, Affoo, & Martin, 2015; Marik, 2001). Pneumonia is the fifth leading cause of infectious death in individuals aged 65 and older and the third leading cause of infectious death in individuals aged 85 and older (LaCroix, Lipson, Miles, & White, 1989). Despite the fact that patients with hyposalivation and xerostomia frequently report symptoms of dysphagia (Dirix, Nuyts, Vander Poorten, Delaere, & Van den Bogaert, 2008; Kuten et al., 1986; Poisson, Laffond, Campos, Dupuis, & Bourdel-Marchasson, 2016; Rogus-Pulia & Logemann, 2011), the role of saliva in the process of swallowing is complex and is not currently well understood.

ORAL HEALTH

The oral health of an individual is defined as "a state of being free of mouth and facial pain, oral and throat cancer, oral infection and sores, birth defects such as cleft lip and palate, periodontal disease, tooth decay and tooth loss, and other diseases and disorders that limit an individual's capacity in biting, chewing, smiling, speaking, and psychological wellbeing" (Petersen & World Health Organization Oral Health Programme, 2003). As mentioned in Chapter 3, saliva plays a critical role in maintaining oral health including (a) protecting the oral mucosa, (b) reducing demineralization and facilitating remineralization of teeth, and (c) sustaining a balanced oral biome and facilitating antimicrobial actions and clearance of pathogens (Humphrey & Williamson, 2001). The relationship between oral health and overall health is complex; however, links between poor oral health and oral preparatory and oral stage dysphagia (Liedberg & Owall, 1991), malnutrition (Daly, Elsner, Allen, & Burke, 2003; Poisson et al., 2016), aspiration pneumonia (Langmore et al., 1998), and increased mortality from pneumonia (Awano et al., 2008) have been documented. It is likely that saliva is a key component of these inter-relationships between oral health, swallowing function, nutritional health, and respiratory health. Figure 6-1 represents a proposed model of the relationship between reduced salivary flow, poor oral health, dysphagia, and suboptimal outcomes.

SECRETIONS AS A PHYSICAL BARRIER TO PATHOGENS

Spinnbarkeit is known to be a structure that promotes lubrication of the oral cavity and pharynx. It also serves as a mucosal barrier that repels colonization of unwanted microbiota with both antifungal and antibacterial effects.

Oral flora is diverse, with a typical healthy individual harboring approximately 700 different bacterial species (Preza, Olsen, Willumsen, Grinde, & Paster, 2009). Although healthy people have fairly uniform bacterial populations throughout their oral cavity, with the microbiome bacteria diversity differs much more between individuals than within a single individual over time. There appear to be site-specific collections that are unique to individuals. Preza et al. (2009) found that the tongue dorsum, cheek, hard palate, and gingiva were sites that were specific for clusters of unique

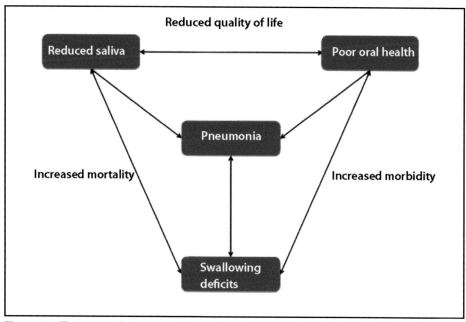

Figure 6-1. The proposed model of the relationship between reduced salivary flow, poor oral health, dysphagia, and suboptimal outcomes.

colonization. Although not fully understood, it is purported that sites within the oral cavity offer differing conditions that lead to the adherence of specific species. Some surfaces favor adherence by specific bacteria that are perhaps less affected by the shear forces of mastication. Others provide safe crevices and resting places that are less affected by salivary flow.

Most pathogens are cleared along with the volume of flowing secretions as swallowing occurs. There is also an active process provided by secretory immunoglobulins that seek and then bind with certain pathogens before adherence to oral mucosa or tooth surfaces occur. Many components of the whole saliva act in a coordinated way to suppress enzyme production in pathogens that break down spinnbarkeit, preventing further adherence to oral and pharyngeal surfaces (Scannapieco, Amin, Salme, & Tezal, 2017; Scannapieco, Torres, & Levine, 1993).

The lung microbiome is constantly seeded by bacteria from the oral cavity in healthy individuals. This can occur during sleep when clearance of secretions is suppressed (Lear, Catz, Grossman, Flanagan, & Moorrees, 1965), during incidental inhalation of airborne pathogens, or during microaspiration of oral pathogens while awake. Bacteria, following arrival into the lungs, are physically moved back out of the lungs by mechanical clearance mechanisms. The mucociliary escalator is one of the mechanisms and covers most of the bronchi and bronchioles. It is made up of a sticky layer of gel-like mucous that traps invasive microorganisms. After trapping, antibodies and macrophages in the mucous identify and destroy invasive organisms. The sticky gel layer, which has collected and bundled the targeted organisms, lies above the ciliated epithelium, which is lined with microscopic, hairlike cilia that rhythmically beat, transporting the organisms via the bronchial airway and trachea to the pharynx where they are either swallowed or expectorated. Healthy lungs are usually cleared through this escalator of newly arrived organisms and particulate within 24 hours.

In a study of 15 healthy volunteers using genetic sequencing of microbes found in the lungs, it was found that bacteria move in and are removed but do not reproduce a great deal (Dickson et al., 2017). It was postulated that in people with damaged lungs (e.g., those with chronic obstructive pulmonary disease and associated poorer clearance mechanisms), the ecosystem is much more hospitable for the reproduction of bacteria.

Xerostomia and Swallowing

As discussed previously in this text, xerostomia is the perception of oral dryness. Xerostomia should not be used synonymously with hyposalivation because these two conditions do not always co-occur; in fact, patients with xerostomia may not have objective signs of hyposalivation (Fox, Busch, & Baum, 1987; Wiener et al., 2010). It is not currently clear why some patients may complain of xerostomia in the presence of adequate salivary volume in the mouth. It is unknown what percentage of the mucosal area must be dry before a patient experiences the sensation of dry mouth (Dawes, 1987). Dawes (1987) hypothesized that because saliva may not be evenly distributed throughout the mouth, it is possible that a focal area of dryness might result in the sensation of oral dryness regardless of the volume of saliva in the oral cavity.

Persons with xerostomia may complain of cracked lips; glossitis; dental caries; oral candidiasis; dry buccal mucosa; burning mouth; halitosis; abnormal taste perception; and difficulty swallowing, speaking, and chewing (Cassolato & Turnbull, 2003). It is not always clear whether the symptoms of xerostomia are related to salivary gland dysfunction or if the symptoms may occur in the absence of salivary gland dysfunction. In a study of patients with head and neck cancer receiving radiotherapy, swallowing complaints such as "food sticking in the mouth," "food sticking in the throat," "needing water to assist with swallowing," and "change in taste" were observed to increase 3 months after radiotherapy. The frequency of these complaints did not appear to be related with saliva production (Logemann et al., 2001). Conversely, Hughes and colleagues (1987) reported a highly significant relationship between stimulated salivary flow rates and subjective complaints of swallowing dysfunction.

Conditions Associated With Xerostomia

Decreased salivary flow, or hyposalivation, results in profound deterioration of oral homeostasis. Increased susceptibility to dental caries and infections, decreased regulation and control of the oral microflora, and impaired swallowing may occur (Sreebny & Vissink, 2010). Salivary gland hypofunction can be caused by developmental or congenital disorders (Eveson, 2008), increased medication usage (Sreebny & Schwartz, 1997), systemic disorders, such as Sjögren's syndrome (Fox & Saito, 2011; Fox, Stern, & Michelson, 2000), radiotherapy-induced damage to salivary acinar tissue (Henson, Inglehart, Eisbruch, & Ship, 2001), and anxiety (Bergdahl & Bergdahl, 2000). Additionally, age-related decreases of whole and submandibular/sublingual salivary flow rates have been reported (Affoo, Foley, Garrick, Siqueira, & Martin, 2015), and decreases of submandibular/sublingual and parotid salivary gland flow rates have been reported in the context of certain diseases, such as Alzheimer's disease (Ship, DeCarli, Friedland, & Baum, 1990; Ship & Puckett, 1994). As discussed previously, hyposalivation does not always result in xerostomia, and xerostomia does not always occur in individuals with hyposalivation. The following discussion includes conditions in which hyposalivation and/or xerostomia are commonly reported as associated symptoms.

Age-Related Decreases of Salivary Flow

An age-related 20% to 40% decrease in the volume of cells responsible for saliva secretion and a corresponding increase of fatty and fibrous tissue in the glandular area have been reported (Baum, 1989; Scott, 1977; Scott, Flower, & Burns, 1987; Sreebny, 2000). Comparable changes have been described for the labial minor glands (Drummond & Chisholm, 1984; Syrjänen & Syrjänen, 1984). This evidence of age-related salivary gland degeneration suggests that functional reductions of salivary flow may also occur. A meta-analysis examining the effect of age on salivary flow rates revealed a significant difference between the whole and submandibular/sublingual salivary flow rates of older and younger adults. A moderate decrease of 0.168 mL/min was identified for the unstimulated whole salivary flow rate, a small decrease of 0.293 mL/min was identified for the stimulated whole salivary flow rate, a moderate decrease of 0.015 mL/min was identified for the unstimulated submandibular/sublingual salivary flow rate, and a moderate decrease of 0.040 mL/min was identified for the stimulated submandibular/sublingual salivary flow rate. The clinical relevance of the finding that whole and submandibular/sublingual salivary flow rates decrease with increasing age remains unknown. Submandibular/sublingual saliva contains mucins (primarily MUC5B and MUC7), which are much less dense in parotid saliva (Amerongen & Veerman, 2002), that contribute to the oral biofilm, a slimy, viscoelastic coating of all surfaces in the oral cavity. The biofilm acts as an important lubricant between opposing oral surfaces during mastication, swallowing, and speaking. Theoretically, age-related reductions of submandibular/sublingual salivary flow rates could contribute to an increased risk of oral infection, inflammation, mechanical wear, and xerostomia and difficulty with speaking, mastication, and swallowing.

Sjögren's Syndrome

Sjögren's syndrome is a chronic, systemic autoimmune disease of the exocrine glands with a typical focal lymphocytic infiltration potentially leading to dry mouth and dry eyes (Kassan & Moutsopoulos, 2004). Primary Sjögren's syndrome occurs when the condition exists as a primary entity, but when it occurs with other autoimmune disorders, it is termed secondary Sjögren's syndrome (Fox & Saito, 2011). Sjögren's syndrome is one of the most prevalent autoimmune diseases, with an estimated 0.5 to 3 million people affected in the United States (Helmick et al., 2008). Individuals with Sjögren's syndrome commonly report symptoms of dysphagia (Rhodus, Colby, et al., 1995; Rhodus, Moller, et al., 1995). Given the prevalence of subjective complaints, several studies have investigated swallowing in individuals with Sjögren's syndrome and confirmed salivary gland dysfunction. Results from this work have indicated that individuals with Sjögren's syndrome complete significantly fewer dry and water bolus swallows compared with healthy control participants (Rhodus, Colby, et al., 1995), and those dry and water bolus swallows may be significantly longer in duration (Caruso, Sonies, Atkinson, & Fox, 1989; Rhodus, Colby, et al., 1995). Rogus-Pulia and Logemann (2011) observed delayed pharyngeal swallow with a cookie bolus and reduced tongue base retraction with a paste and cookie bolus in a group of individuals with Sjögren's syndrome. Durational measures such as the time for the base of the tongue to come into contact with the posterior pharyngeal wall were observed to be prolonged when the boluses were smaller and thinner. Additionally, the laryngeal closure to cricopharyngeal opening measure was longer for thicker-consistency boluses than for thinner-consistency boluses. A significantly larger amount of oral and pharyngeal residue was found for those with Sjögren's syndrome, and there were significantly more occurrences of laryngeal penetration. A significant, positive correlation was observed between the oral transit time and the salivary flow rate for 5 mL of thin liquid. A significant negative correlation was found between the pharyngeal response time and the salivary flow rate for paste.

Head and Neck Cancer Treatment

Head and neck cancer accounts for 3% of malignancies in the United States, translating to approximately 63,000 Americans developing head and neck cancer annually (Siegel, Miller, & Jemal, 2017). Radiotherapy is commonly used to treat head and neck cancer; however, this form of treatment is associated with a number of acute and long-term side effects, including salivary gland dysfunction. Xerostomia is another common complication of radiotherapy for head and neck cancer (Dirix et al., 2008). There is a substantial body of literature dedicated to examining the impact of head and neck cancer and the treatment of head and neck cancer on the safety and efficiency of swallowing.

Salivary glands are significantly impacted by radiation with high levels of cell death observed within a few days or weeks of radiotherapy (Hall, Robinson, & Green, 2000). Salivary glands are composed of slowly proliferating, highly differentiated cells, and cellular death results in a reduced volume of secretion in addition to altered composition. Due to the fact that salivary gland cells are slow to proliferate, individuals who undergo radiotherapy may experience salivary gland dysfunction for months or even years after treatment (Dirix et al., 2008; Eisbruch et al., 2001; Li, Taylor, Ten Haken, & Eisbruch, 2007). Some individuals may even experience permanent salivary gland hypofunction (Li et al., 2007). Studies that have specifically examined swallowing in individuals who have experienced radiotherapy-induced damage to salivary acinar tissue report an increase in subjective complaints related to dry mouth. There may be a relationship between the quantity of saliva and the oral transit time, pharyngeal swallow delay, and degree of oropharyngeal stasis (Logemann et al., 2001; Rogus-Pulia et al., 2016). In addition to these problems, radiation therapy also increases the rate of development of tooth decay, largely due to the reduction in calcium secreted by damaged salivary glands. The effect of tooth loss on the efficiency of mastication and the associated reduction in the range of foods that may be consumed due to edentulism have a great impact on nutrition and quality of life.

Newer techniques for treating head and neck cancers such as intensity-modulated radiation therapy (IMRT) allow for more discrete treatment of cancerous lesions. Careful delivery of the radiation beam now allows for reductions in exposure to the salivary glands with a presumed decrease in rates of xerostomia. In a study of patients undergoing parotid-sparing IMRT by Richards and colleagues (2017), it was found that there were decreases in both the volume and composition of salivary production in the 3- to 6-month period after the initiation of radiation therapy. However, after 12 months, there were fewer significant differences in these measures, indicating good functional recovery with this technique. Interestingly, patients with high-grade xerostomia in this study had lower rates of total protein output at 12 months after treatment. In particular, there was a reduction in the secretion of calcium in patients with sustained high-grade xerostomia. Calcium is believed to contribute to the linking of mucins to form spinnbarkeit along the buccal mucosal surface (Raynal, Hardingham, Sheehan, & Thornton, 2003).

Lal et al. (2018) performed a prospective study in patients receiving IMRT and assessed the salivary flow rate and the subjective perception of dryness and stickiness with objective saliva flow measurements before and after radiotherapy. It was again found that decreases in salivary flow were associated with xerostomia, but they largely resolved after 12 months with the sparing of the parotid glands during radiotherapy. This translated into objective and subjective improvement of both xerostomia and quality of life scores at the close of the study; however, the subjective score for sticky saliva did not improve with salivary flow. The authors suggested that alterations in submandibular and/or sublingual gland function may have the greatest impact on the sensation of stickiness because the mucins are not found in the parotid secretions in as great a number as in the other glands. Although calcium production from the parotid may play a large role in the prevention of xerostomia as well as its protective role in preventing tooth decay in patients undergoing radiation treatment, it may not be enough to offset the symptom of sticky saliva.

There are anticipatory actions that can be taken after a diagnosis of head and neck cancer that include encouragement to increase oral hygiene measures and guidance to eliminate or reduce high-risk behaviors including smoking and alcohol consumption. This may require the engagement of an interdisciplinary team of physicians, nurses, dentists, speech-language pathologists, and others that can attend to psychosocial needs of the patient. Radiation-induced xerostomia and mucosal ulcerations increase the risk of viral, bacterial, and fungal infections. Attention should be directed to the continued use of ill-fitting dentures because the fit may change with weight loss, and ulcerations will be more difficult to treat in the setting of radiation toxicity. Oral candidiasis is a common opportunistic fungal infection that is often found following radiation treatment as a result of a disequilibrium of the oral biome. Patients may present with white, patchy lesions or red diffused lesions on the oral mucosa. During radiation therapy, oral candidiasis is often mistaken as oropharyngeal mucositis and may be accompanied by burning and pain (Wong, 2013). The treatment is usually an oral antifungal agent that is swished and expectorated or swished and swallowed such as fluconazole, ketoconazole, and itraconazole (Clarkson, Worthington, & Eden, 2007). Other treatments can range from simple toothbrushing and the use of salivary substitutes to the recent development of cutting-edge techniques using stem cells to regenerate salivary secretory cells (Tanaka et al., 2018).

Alzheimer's Disease

It has been estimated that 32% to 93% of patients with Alzheimer's disease suffer from dysphagia (Affoo, Foley, Rosenbek, Shoemaker, & Martin, 2013; Feinberg, Ekberg, Segall, & Tully, 1992; Volicer et al., 1989). Currently, more than 5.8 million Americans are living with Alzheimer's disease or another dementia, and, by 2050, this number could increase to as many as 14 million (Alzheimer's Association, 2019). Compared with the mortality rates of diseases such as heart disease and cancer, which have decreased since the year 2000, deaths from Alzheimer's disease have increased by 145%, and, currently, 1 out of every 3 older adults dies from Alzheimer's disease or another dementia (Alzheimer's Association, 2019).

Instrumental assessment of swallowing in persons with Alzheimer's disease has revealed deficits of the oral and pharyngeal stages of swallowing (Feinberg et al., 1992; Garon, Sierzant, & Ormiston, 2009; Horner, Alberts, Dawson, & Cook, 1994; Humbert, McLaren, Malandraki, Johnson, & Robbins, 2011; Humbert et al., 2010; Priefer & Robbins, 1997; Suh, Kim, & Na, 2009; Wada et al., 2001). Oral deficits include prolonged bolus preparation and oral transit times. Pharyngeal deficits include delayed pharyngeal swallow initiation, reduced hyolaryngeal excursion, laryngeal penetration, tracheal aspiration, and pharyngeal residue after swallowing. Autonomic nervous system dysfunction has been reported in individuals with Alzheimer's disease (Affoo et al., 2013), and it has been hypothesized that autonomic nervous system dysfunction could contribute to the presence of dysphagia in this population. Resting and stimulated submandibular salivary flow has been reported to be reduced in unmedicated individuals with mild Alzheimer's disease (Ship et al., 1990). Forty-six percent of a sample of individuals with Alzheimer's disease had flow rates below the tenth percentile compared with 11% of a healthy age-matched control group. Despite these findings, no studies have been undertaken that explore the relationship between hyposalivation and swallowing. Additionally, due to the cognitive impairments associated with Alzheimer's disease, this population may not be able to communicate feelings of perceived oral dryness.

Aspiration Pneumonia

Aspiration pneumonia is a lung infection that is acquired when an offending substance, such as food/liquid, secretions, or regurgitated contents of the stomach or esophagus, enters the lungs. It is often presumed that misdirection of food, liquid, or secretions into the lungs in a patient with disordered swallowing is the essential predisposing element for the development of aspiration pneumonia. Aspiration pneumonia is globally considered a major cause of morbidity and mortality. Langmore and colleagues (1998) were the first to draw a connection between the condition of the oral cavity and the advent of aspiration pneumonia. Although dysphagia was concluded to be an important risk for aspiration pneumonia, it was not sufficient to cause pneumonia unless other risk factors were present. In that study, dependence for oral care and the number of decayed teeth were among the strongest predictors for pneumonia. This was a revelation at the time of publication, and this research generated considerable interest in the study of the oral biome and its contribution to associated pneumonias.

As previously discussed, humans are constantly aspirating microscopic airborne pathogens and particulate into the lower airways. Research suggests that microaspiration of food and liquid is a normal event that a healthy person can tolerate (Butler et al., 2014). It is assumed that a combination of good oral health, good oral clearance, good airway clearance, and a robust immune response from the body when encountering foreign material in the airway are key elements in our ability to tolerate these aspiration events. However, during episodes of impaired health, these elements are not ensured.

The fluid characteristics of saliva are indispensable for the mechanical rinsing of the oral cavity. We know that movement of saliva through the oral cavity is important for dissolving taste substances and transporting them to taste receptor sites, but saliva is also important in protection of the mucosa, food bolus formation, clearance of food debris, and microorganisms. The movement of microorganisms from the oral cavity is very important to sustaining oral health. When epithelial cells of the oral mucosa die and are sloughed off of the mucosal layer, saliva plays an important role in the clearance of these cells from the oral cavity. Each cell can carry approximately 100 different microorganisms (Dawes, 2003). The microorganisms can populate a single milliliter of saliva with approximately 100 million bacterial cells. If we consider that normal salivary flow is more or less 750 mL/day, we begin to realize the volume of organic biota that needs to be shed. It is estimated that approximately 5 to 10 g bacterial cells are cleared from the oral cavity in a normal adult with good salivary flow (Curtis, Zenobia, & Darveau, 2011). This constant flushing of dead cells and the very alive microbiota through salivary flow and subsequent swallowing is essential to sustaining good oral health (Kolenbrander, Palmer, Periasamy, & Jakubovics, 2010). The mucins in the saliva continue to adhere to tooth and mucosal surfaces and promote continued colonization of much of the good bacteria that is flushed with swallowing. In this way, the normal microbiome is sustained. When salivary flow is impaired, the flushing of the dead cells and the associated microorganisms becomes impaired. Less saliva also results in gaps in the equilibrium of the oral biome with dry spots becoming host to species that are without a healthy population to contain their growth.

The mechanisms of airway clearance are impaired in many disease processes. The mucociliary escalator can be inhibited by smoking, which causes paralysis of the movement of the cilia, chronic respiratory diseases, changes in the character of the mucous, and dehydration. When the microbiota of the oral cavity is mixed with food, liquid, or secretions and aspirated into the lungs, the process for removing begins rather quickly. If the pathogens are allowed to rest in the lungs, certain bacteria can thrive and reproduce, resulting in a larger and less diverse population than is found in the oral cavity with an increase in the offending bacterial population, consolidation of the new colony, and, if the immune response is poor, a resulting infection.

In a study by El-Solh and colleagues (2004), oral plaques were collected from critically ill patients requiring intensive care treatment. The samples were examined, and the biome was identified using genetic sequencing techniques. Following this, bronchial alveolar lavage was performed to collect samples of the biome from the lung with a finding of matching pathogens in both the oral cavity and lungs. It is now accepted that there is a strong relationship between poor oral health and respiratory disease.

Ventilator Dependence, Xerostomia, and Pneumonia

It is well known that patients undergoing mechanical ventilation via an endotracheal tube are at risk of ventilator-associated pneumonia (VAP). The prevalence rate of VAP in patients undergoing mechanical ventilation is 9% to 68% (Gatell et al., 2012), and it is the second most prevalent cause of nosocomial pneumonia with mortality rates reported between 30% and 70% (Micik et al., 2013). It is costly in that it increases the length of mechanical ventilation with resulting increases in morbidity, mortality, and patient distress (Craven, Lei, Ruthazer, Sarwar, & Hudcova, 2013).

Patients with endotracheal tubes experience a decline in oral health. This decline can be exacerbated by the presence of malnutrition, orogastric tubes with associated derangements of hydration, and changes in salivation caused by constant mouth opening, fever, diarrhea, and analgesia. Mouth opening from transoral endotracheal and/or orogastric tubes is particularly problematic because they not only cause the mouth to remain open and go dry but also make oral care difficult (Haghighi, Shafipour, Bagheri-Nesami, Gholipour Baradari, & Yazdani Charati, 2017). Patients in intensive care units on ventilation form dental plaques that appear more quickly and in greater volumes than in other patient populations (Hutchins, Karras, Erwin, & Sullivan, 2009). The oral biome

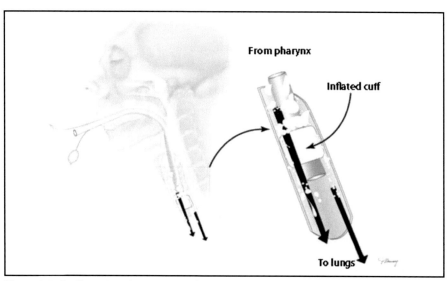

Figure 6-2. An illustration showing an endotracheal tube placed transorally and into the tracheal airway. Although a properly inflated cuff will keep most from traveling into the lower airways, some secretions and debris can enter into the lower lung fields. (Reprinted with permission from Joseph Murray, PhD, CCC-SLP, BCS-S.)

changes in the first 2 days after hospitalization with greater colonization of Gram-negative organisms in dental plaques (Kaya et al., 2017), which when combined with saliva and aspirated into the lungs are known causes of VAP (Hillier, Wilson, Chamberlain, & King, 2013).

The aspiration of pathogens into the lungs in this patient population is assumed, but the mechanism for these events is not well studied. Intuitively, the presence of an endotracheal tube in the oral cavity would obstruct the propulsive components of the swallow. For instance, tongue base retraction will be incomplete in contact with the posterior pharyngeal wall, preventing envelopment of any secretions in the oral cavity and pharynx and resulting in poor interbolus pressures. The sequelae to this would be a disruption in the transport of the secretions and retention of these same secretions in the collecting cavities of the oral cavity, valleculae, and pyriform sinuses in the distal pharynx. As the volume of the secretions increase, the capacity of the collecting cavities to contain the secretions will be challenged and will eventually fail with transport of the secretions into the open tracheal lumen along the endotracheal tube. Even cuffed endotracheal tubes cannot prevent the travel of microorganisms into the lower airways (Figure 6-2).

When secretions containing these pathogens arrive in the lungs, they set off a signal to the body that an infection is occurring, with the body responding with the release of white blood cells to fight the colonization. It is now understood that feedback loops can occur between the bacteria and immune defenses. Some pathogens grow faster when exposed to these signals from the body to produce white blood cells. The increased growth of the invading biome causes increased inflammation, which then triggers more signals to produce white blood cells. This looping interaction is either advanced to the point of inflammation and infection, resulting in pneumonia, or terminated with a combination of immune response and dislocation of the offending pathogens through mucociliary elevation (Dickson et al., 2015).

Oral Care and Pneumonia

Interventions were developed to reduce the risk of aspiration by suppressing the growth of pathogens in the oral biome through the provision of oral care. It was soon determined through controlled study and randomly controlled trials and then verified through meta-analysis that oral care did in fact result in a reduction in the occurrence of VAP in intensive care units (Longti & Zheng, 2015; Munro & Grap, 2004). One study showed that the implementation of an oral care program in intensive care units could significantly decrease the relative risk of VAP and the prevalence from 10.4 to 3.9 cases per 1000 ventilator days (Fields, 2008).

The assurance of provision of oral care is difficult to achieve, particularly in frail older adults most at risk of pneumonia. Some afflictions of older adults that can lead to inadequate oral health include cognitive impairment (Arai, Sumi, Uematsu, & Miura, 2003), functional disability (Hawkins, 1999), and decreased hand function (Padilha, Hugo, Hilgert, & Dal Moro, 2007). In institutionalized settings, the loss of functional ability and autonomy may create a barrier to performing oral hygiene self-care and can constrain access to professional oral health care. Sarcopenia and generalized weakness from the synergy of multiple comorbidities may also contribute to reduced quality and quantity of oral care that is self-administered.

A typical care routine might include elevation of the head of the bed from 30 to 45 degrees and the use of a swab and chlorhexidine 0.2% solution every 12 hours by nurses. However, other simpler care can also have a therapeutic and preventative effect in both ventilated and nonventilated patients. Kaneoka et al. (2015) performed a systematic review and meta-analysis that showed a significant risk reduction in pneumonia through oral care interventions. The effects of mechanical oral care (toothbrushing) alone showed risk reduction for fatal pneumonia.

Liu and colleagues (2018) published a Cochrane review of oral care measures for the prophylaxis of aspiration pneumonia in the nursing home population. In that review, several methods for delivery were cited from the National Institute for Health and Care Excellence guidelines. The nature of oral care measures that have been proposed is described as being diverse. They can be classified as follows (Liu et al., 2018):

- Mechanical aids to remove plaque and debris from the oral cavity
  - Toothbrushing
  - Swabbing with water
- Topical (chemical) disinfection to reduce colonization
  - Mouth rinses
  - Sprays
  - Liquids
  - Gels
  - Antiseptics
    - Saline
    - Chlorhexidine
    - Povidone-iodine
- Combination of mechanical plaque removal and topical disinfection
  - Swabbing with antiseptic
  - Toothbrushing with antibacterial toothpaste
  - Daily toothbrushing plus antiseptic rinse
- Professional dental care:
  - Aided toothbrushing
  - Suction to remove excess fluid

ASSESSMENT

The diagnosis of salivary gland dysfunction requires a comprehensive dental and medical evaluation, including the assessment of salivary output (Navazesh, Christensen, & Brightman, 1992). However, xerostomia is the perception of oral dryness and may occur with or without salivary dysfunction (Navazesh & Ship, 1983). Assessment for the purposes of detecting xerostomia should then focus on patient-reported outcome measures (PROMs), which are instruments that report the status of a patient's health condition based on reports directly from the patient. One such tool, the 8-item visual analog scale (VAS) xerostomia questionnaire (Pai, Ghezzi, & Ship, 2001), was developed using healthy participants with no systemic or salivary diseases who were not taking prescription or antihistamine medications. The xerostomia questionnaire was administered at baseline and, for a subgroup of participants, after salivary perturbation. Results indicated that nearly all the VAS items showed significant reliability; however, the VAS items had poor to moderate validity when they were compared with objective salivary flow measures at baseline. A moving average measure was calculated and found to improve data analyses by controlling variability in VAS and salivary flow measures over a 6-hour period. Although these findings suggest that it may not be possible to identify salivary gland dysfunction using the 8-item VAS xerostomia questionnaire, this tool can certainly aid a clinician in identifying the presence of xerostomia, and it may also be possible to document changes over time.

The Xerostomia Inventory is a validated PROM composed of questions related to oral dryness in which patients rate their responses on a 5-point ordinal scale (Thomson, Chalmers, Spencer, & Williams, 1999). Another PROM that may be used to evaluate dryness is the Clinical Oral Dryness Score, which was designed to objectively assess and quantify oral dryness by visually inspecting the oral cavity and documenting clinical signs of oral dryness (Challacombe & Osailan, 2015; Osailan, Pramanik, Shirlaw, Proctor, & Challacombe, 2012). Items include such observations as "mirror sticks to buccal mucosa and "mirror sticks to tongue," which could be easily incorporated into a clinical evaluation. It has been suggested that this objective measure may be a useful adjunct to self-report in the assessment of xerostomia and/or salivary dysfunction (Jager, Bots, Forouzanfar, & Brand, 2018).

TREATMENT

Saliva Stimulation and Swallowing

The treatment of xerostomia can fall into one of two categories, treatment focused on alleviating the perception of dry mouth or treatment focused on stimulating the salivary flow rate in order to increase the volume of saliva in the mouth. The following discussion first addresses treatments focused on alleviating the perception of dry mouth followed by treatments meant to stimulate salivary secretion.

Saliva substitutes come in the form of oral sprays, gels, and mouthwashes and are available over the counter. These products have been found to alleviate xerostomia temporarily (Skrinjar et al., 2015). Depending on the active ingredients, some products have also been reported to stimulate salivary secretion. A comprehensive review of these products and their effects can be found in Chapters 5 and 8. Saliva substitutes and oral moisturizers have also been found to impact swallowing in two studies. Rogus-Pulia and colleagues (2018) examined perceptions of swallowing effort before and after the application of Biotene Oral Balance Moisturizing Gel in healthy older adults. They found that perceived mouth dryness was associated with greater perceived swallowing effort and that swallowing effort decreased significantly after the application of Biotene Oral Balance Moisturizing Gel. Rhodus and Bereuter (2000) evaluated the effects of a commercially available oral moisturizer on the salivary flow rate, symptoms of xerostomia, oral pH, oral microflora, and swallowing in nine postirradiation patients with head and neck cancer, six patients with primary Sjögren's syndrome, and nine patients with secondary Sjögren's syndrome. They reported that after the use of an oral moisturizer for 2 weeks, whole unstimulated salivary flow rates were observed to be significantly improved compared with baseline. Additionally, swallowing both subjectively and objectively improved in 75% of patients. The pharyngeal transit time was found to be decreased by 0.5 seconds in the study population.

Intraoral electrostimulation had been explored as a method of stimulating salivary secretion and alleviating symptoms of xerostomia (Strietzel et al., 2011). This technique showed a significant improvement in the short term (3 months) in symptoms such as frequency and severity of dryness and difficulty swallowing and in the long term (5 months) in symptoms such as frequency and severity of dryness, oral discomfort, difficulty in sleeping and talking, and the rate of unstimulated salivary secretion.

Several studies have examined the use of acupuncture to treat xerostomia and hyposalivation (Blom & Lundeberg, 2000; Cohen, Menter, & Hale, 2005; Rydholm & Strang, 1999); however, a recent systematic review of these studies and others found that the current evidence is insufficient to conclude whether acupuncture is an effective treatment option for xerostomia and/or hyposalivation (Assy & Brand, 2018).

Traditional and complementary medicine in the form of Chinese herbal treatments have also been trialed as an adjunct to conventional cancer treatment. Researchers using Chinese medicine consider the effect of radiotherapy as a heat toxin that injures body fluid with resulting symptoms of oral dryness, mucositis, poor appetite, lethargy, and insomnia (Lim et al., 2019). The remedies studied have included herbs Sha Shen Mai Dong Tang and Gan Lu Yin, and systematic reviews suggest that these Chinese herbal treatments may lessen xerostomia (Nik Nabil, Lim, Chan, Lai, & Liew, 2018; Park, Noh, & Choi, 2018), oral mucositis, and anorexia associated with radiotherapy. It is proposed that the mechanism for promoting salivary fluid secretion (Wei & Yongming, 2009) is achieved by activating receptors to increase calcium and stimulation of transporters for chloride (Murakami, Wei, Ding, & Zhang, 2009). Another herb, Tian Hua Fen, is thought to "clear heat" and stimulate body fluid secretion (Arawwawala, Thabrew, Arambewela, & Handunnetti, 2010). It is also known to possess anti-inflammatory effects, which may inhibit mucositis related to radiotherapy (Park et al., 2018).

Some studies have documented that increased oral cavity stimulation is associated with increased salivary secretion. Salivary secretion increases with the hardness and the size of an object being chewed as well as the forces generated by the chewing muscles (Anderson & Hector, 1987; Hector & Linden, 1987; Rosenhek, Macpherson, & Dawes, 1993; Yeh et al., 2000). Increased saliva secretion has also been reported after the application of vibration stimuli to the facial skin overlying the bilateral belly of the masseter muscles, possibly due to the tonic vibration reflex resulting in contraction of the masseter muscles and/or the vibration activating various types of mechanoreceptors through the skin and mucosa (Hiraba, Yamaoka, Fukano, Fujiwara, & Ueda, 2008).

The use of toothbrushing as a mechanical form of whole salivary flow stimulation has been examined previously in healthy young adults (Hoek, Brand, Veerman, & Amerongen, 2002; Ligtenberg, Brand, Bots, & Nieuw Amerongen, 2006), in older adults free of systemic disease (Affoo et al., 2018), and in older adults with clinically significant hyposalivation (Papas et al., 2006). Salivary flow increases lasting from 5 to 60 minutes have been reported (Affoo et al., 2018; Hoek et al., 2002; Ligtenberg et al., 2006; Papas et al., 2006), which would be expected to contribute to the oral biofilm in the mouth, promoting optimal oral homeostasis and potentially increasing oral comfort. Increasing the salivary volume may also affect salivary clearance in that the volume of oral saliva contributes to triggering of the pharyngeal stage of swallowing (Dawes, 1983), in addition to increasing the rate of swallowing (Lagerlöf & Dawes, 1984).

Evidence suggests that very simple and readily available solutions may provide longer-lasting relief (Assery, 2019). A study of 54 patients complaining of a sensation of dry mouth compared artificial saliva, 3% citric acid, and distilled water. Fifteen minutes after the solution intake, 12 patients (67%) belonging to the artificial saliva group, 9 (50%) from the citric acid group, and 2 (11%) from the water group reported significant symptomatologic improvement. After 1 hour of solution intake, 7 patients (39%) from the artificial saliva group, 10 (56%) from the citric acid group, and 0 from the water group noted significant symptomatologic improvement.

The importance of saliva in sustaining whole-body health cannot be overstated. As has been reviewed in this chapter, saliva has numerous components that function to facilitate sensation, gustation, bolus manipulation, and eventual safe and efficient transport of food and liquid to the lower enteral tract. The same mucins in saliva that contribute to lubrication and taste sensation provide protective functions by simultaneously harboring a vast and varied oral biome while suppressing the growth of pathogens and creating a barrier between the biome and the host tissue and bloodstream. We know that a reduction in the volume of saliva can lead to a derangement of the oral biome that can lead to dramatic systemic infections, such as aspiration pneumonia, but also more insidious, long-term problems in oral discomfort during mastication, including loss of taste and declination in swallow function that can have a synergistic effect on the overall health and quality of life of the individual. The collective effect of hyposalivation can lead to a decline in nutrition with an associated decline in function that combines in an interwoven spiral of ill health and the inability to recover from health-related stressors. Interventions to address hyposalivation, both old and new, are known to have a beneficial effect on oral health. There is warranted optimism that continued investigation into the wide-ranging and varied interventions will result in improved overall health and quality of life for those individuals suffering from hyposalivation.

REFERENCES

Affoo, R. H., Foley, N., Garrick, R., Siqueira, W. L., & Martin, R. E. (2015). Meta-analysis of salivary flow rates in young and older adults. *Journal of the American Geriatric Society, 63*(10), 2142-2151. doi:10.1111/jgs.13652

Affoo, R. H., Foley, N., Rosenbek, J., Shoemaker, J. K., & Martin, R. E. (2013). Swallowing dysfunction and autonomic nervous system dysfunction in Alzheimer's disease: A scoping review of the evidence. *Journal of the American Geriatric Society, 61*(12), 2203-2213. doi:10.1111/jgs.12553

Affoo, R. H., Trottier, K., Garrick, R., Mascarenhas, T., Jang, Y., & Martin, R. E. (2018). The effects of tooth brushing on whole salivary flow rate in older adults. *Biomed Research International, 2018*, 3904139. doi:10.1155/2018/3904139

Alzheimer's Association. (2019). Alzheimer's disease facts and figures. *Alzheimer's & Dementia, 15*(3), 321-387. doi:10.1016/j.jalz.2019.01.010.

Amerongen, A. V., & Veerman, E. C. (2002). Saliva—The defender of the oral cavity. *Oral Diseases, 8*(1), 12-22. doi:10.1034/j.1601-0825.2002.10816.x

Anderson, D. J., & Hector, M. P. (1987). Periodontal mechanoreceptors and parotid secretion in animals and man. *Journal of Dental Research, 66*(2), 518-523. doi:10.1177/00220345870660022201

Arai, K., Sumi, Y., Uematsu, H., & Miura, H. (2003). Association between dental health behaviours, mental/physical function and self-feeding ability among the elderly: A cross-sectional survey. *Gerodontology, 20*(2), 78-83. doi: 10.1111/j.1741-2358.2003.00078.x

Arawwawala, M., Thabrew, I., Arambewela, L., & Handunnetti, S. (2010). Anti-inflammatory activity of trichosanthes cucumerina Linn. in rats. *Journal of Ethnopharmacology, 131*(3), 538-543. doi:10.1016/j.jep.2010.07.028

Assery, M. K. A. (2019). Efficacy of artificial salivary substitutes in treatment of xerostomia: A systematic review. *Journal of Pharmacy and Bioallied Sciences, 11*(Suppl. 1), S1-S12. doi:10.4103/jpbs.JPBS_220_18

Assy, Z., & Brand, H. S. (2018). A systematic review of the effects of acupuncture on xerostomia and hyposalivation. *BMC Complementary and Alternative Medicine, 18*(1), 57. doi:10.1186/s12906-018-2124-x

Awano, S., Ansai, T., Takata, Y., Soh, I., Akifusa, S., Hamasaki, T., ... Takehara, T. (2008). Oral health and mortality risk from pneumonia in the elderly. *Journal of Dental Research, 87*(4), 334-339. doi:10.1177/154405910808700418

Baum, B. J. (1989). Salivary gland fluid secretion during aging. *Journal of the American Geriatric Society, 37*(5), 453-458. doi:10.1111/j.1532-5415.1989.tb02644.x

Bergdahl, M., & Bergdahl, J. (2000). Low unstimulated salivary flow and subjective oral dryness: Association with medication, anxiety, depression, and stress. *Journal of Dental Research, 79*(9), 1652-1658. doi:10.1177/00220345000790090301

Blom, M., & Lundeberg, T. (2000). Long-term follow-up of patients treated with acupuncture for xerostomia and the influence of additional treatment. *Oral Diseases, 6*(1), 15-24.

Bosma, J. F. (1957). Deglutition: Pharyngeal stage. *Physiological Reviews, 37*(3), 275-300. doi:10.1152/physrev.1957.37.3.275

Butler, S. G., Clark, H., Baginski, S. G., Todd, J. T., Lintzenich, C., & Leng, X. (2014). Computed tomography pulmonary findings in healthy older adult aspirators versus nonaspirators. *Laryngoscope, 124*(2), 494-497. doi:10.1002/lary.24284

Caruso, A. J., Sonies, B. C., Atkinson, J. C., & Fox, P. C. (1989). Objective measures of swallowing in patients with primary Sjögren's syndrome. *Dysphagia, 4*(2), 101-105. doi:10.1007/BF02407153

Cassolato, S. F., & Turnbull, R. S. (2003). Xerostomia: Clinical aspects and treatment. *Gerodontology, 20*(2), 64-77. doi:10.1111/j.1741-2358.2003.00064.x

Challacombe, S., & Osailan, S. (2015). Clinical scoring scales for assessment of dry mouth. In G. Carpenter (Ed.), *Dry mouth: A clinical guide on causes, effects and treatments* (pp. 119-132). Berlin, Germany: Springer.

Clarkson, J. E., Worthington, H. V., & Eden, O. B. (2007). Interventions for treating oral mucositis for patients with cancer receiving treatment. *Cochrane Database of Systematic Reviews, 2*, CD001973. doi:10.1002/14651858.CD001973.pub3

Cohen, A. J., Menter, A., & Hale, L. (2005). Acupuncture: Role in comprehensive cancer care—A primer for the oncologist and review of the literature. *Integrative Cancer Therapies, 4*(2), 131-143. doi:10.1177/1534735405276419

Collins, L. M., & Dawes, C. (1987). The surface area of the adult human mouth and thickness of the salivary film covering the teeth and oral mucosa. *Journal of Dental Research, 66*(8), 1300-1302. doi:10.1177/00220345870660080201

Craven, D. E., Lei, Y., Ruthazer, R., Sarwar, A., & Hudcova, J. (2013). Incidence and outcomes of ventilator-associated tracheobronchitis and pneumonia. *American Journal of Medicine, 126*(6), 542-549. doi:10.1016/j.amjmed.2012.12.012

Curtis, M. A., Zenobia, C., & Darveau, R. P. (2011). The relationship of the oral microbiotia to periodontal health and disease. *Cell Host and Microbe, 10*(4), 302-306. doi:10.1016/j.chom.2011.09.008

Daly, R. M., Elsner, R. J., Allen, P. F., & Burke, F. M. (2003). Associations between self-reported dental status and diet. *Journal of Oral Rehabilitation, 30*(10), 964-970. doi:10.1046/j.1365-2842.2003.01169.x

Dawes, C. (1983). A mathematical model of salivary clearance of sugar from the oral cavity. *Caries Research, 17*(4), 321-334. doi:10.1159/000260684

Dawes, C. (1987). Physiological factors affecting salivary flow rate, oral sugar clearance, and the sensation of dry mouth in man. *Journal of Dental Research, 66*(Spec. No.), 648-653. doi:10.1177/00220345870660S107

Dawes, C. (2003). Estimates, from salivary analyses, of the turnover time of the oral mucosal epithelium in humans and the number of bacteria in an edentulous mouth. *Archives of Oral Biology, 48*(5), 329-336. doi:10.1016/s0003-9969(03)00014-1

Dawes, C., Pedersen, A. M., Villa, A., Ekström, J., Proctor, G. B., Vissink, A., … Wolff, A. (2015). The functions of human saliva: A review sponsored by the World Workshop on Oral Medicine VI. *Archives of Oral Biology, 60*(6), 863-874. doi:10.1016/j.archoralbio.2015.03.004

Dickson, R. P., Erb-Downward, J. R., Freeman, C. M., McCloskey, L., Falkowski, N. R., Huffnagle, G. B., & Curtis, J. L. (2017). Bacterial topography of the healthy human lower respiratory tract. *American Society for Microbiology, 8*(1), e02287-16. doi:10.1128/mBio.02287-16

Dickson, R. P., Erb-Downward, J. R., Prescott, H. C., Martinez, F. J., Curtis, J. L., Lama, V. N., & Huffnagle, G. B. (2015). Intraalveolar catecholamines and the human lung microbiome. *American Journal of Respiratory and Critical Care Medicine, 192*(2), 257-259. doi:10.1164/rccm.201502-0326LE

Dietsch, A. M., Pelletier, C. A., & Solomon, N. P. (2018). Saliva production and enjoyment of real-food flavors in people with and without dysphagia and/or xerostomia. *Dysphagia, 33*(6), 803-808. doi:10.1007/s00455-018-9905-8

Dirix, P., Nuyts, S., Vander Poorten, V., Delaere, P., & Van den Bogaert, W. (2008). The influence of xerostomia after radiotherapy on quality of life: Results of a questionnaire in head and neck cancer. *Support Care in Cancer, 16*(2), 171-179. doi:10.1007/s00520-007-0300-5

Dodds, W. J. (1989). The physiology of swallowing. *Dysphagia, 3*, 171-178. doi:10.1007/BF02407219

Drummond, J. R., & Chisholm, D. M. (1984). A qualitative and quantitative study of the ageing human labial salivary glands. *Archives of Oral Biology, 29*(2), 151-155. doi:10.1016/0003-9969(84)90120-1

Dynesen, A. W. (2015). Oral dryness, dietary intake, and alterations in taste. In G. Carpenter (Ed.), *Dry Mouth* (pp. 69-80). Berlin, Germany: Springer.

Eisbruch, A., Kim, H. M., Terrell, J. E., Marsh, L. H., Dawson, L. A., & Ship, J. A. (2001). Xerostomia and its predictors following parotid-sparing irradiation of head-and-neck cancer. *International Journal of Radiation Oncology • Biology • Physics, 50*(3), 695-704. doi:10.1016/S0360-3016(01)01512-7

El-Solh, A. A., Pietrantoni, C., Bhat, A., Okada, M., Zambon, J., Aquilina, A., & Berbary, E. (2004). Colonization of dental plaques: A reservoir of respiratory pathogens for hospital-acquired pneumonia in institutionalized elders. *Chest, 126*(5), 1575-1582. doi:10.1378/chest.126.5.1575

Eveson, J. W. (2008). Xerostomia. *Periodontology 2000, 48*, 85-91. doi:10.1111/j.1600-0757.2008.00263.x

Feinberg, M. J., Ekberg, O., Segall, L., & Tully, J. (1992). Deglutition in elderly patients with dementia: Findings of videofluorographic evaluation and impact on staging and management. *Radiology, 183*(3), 811-814. doi:10.1148/radiology.183.3.1584939

Fields, L. B. (2008). Oral care intervention to reduce incidence of ventilator-associated pneumonia in the neurologic intensive care unit. *Journal of Neuroscience Nursing, 40*(5), 291-298. doi:10.1097/01376517-200810000-00007

Foley, N. C., Affoo, R. H., & Martin, R. E. (2015). A systematic review and meta-analysis examining pneumonia-associated mortality in dementia. *Dementia and Geriatric Cognitive Disorders, 39*(1-2), 52-67. doi:10.1159/000367783

Fox, P. C., Busch, K. A., & Baum, B. J. (1987). Subjective reports of xerostomia and objective measures of salivary gland performance. *Journal of the American Dental Association, 115*(4), 581-584. doi:10.1016/S0002-8177(87)54012-0

Fox, C. M., & Saito, R. I. (2011). Sjögren's syndrome. In M. Hertl (Ed.), *Autoimmune diseases of the skin: Pathogenesis, diagnosis, management* (pp. 283-324). New York, NY: SpringerWien.

Fox, R. I., Stern, M., & Michelson, P. (2000). Update in Sjögren syndrome. *Current Opinion in Rheumatology, 12*(5), 391-398.

Garon, B. R., Sierzant, T., & Ormiston, C. (2009). Silent aspiration: Results of 2,000 video fluoroscopic evaluations. *Journal of Neuroscience Nursing, 41*(4), 178-185; quiz 186-177. doi:10.1097/JNN.0b013e3181aaaade

Gatell, J., Santé, R. M., Hernández, V. Ó., Carrillo, S. E., Turégano, D. C., Fernández, M. I., & Vallés, D. J. (2012). Assessment of a training programme for the prevention of ventilator-associated pneumonia. *Nursing in Critical Care, 17*(6), 285-292. doi:10.1111/j.1478-5153.2012.00526.x.

Haghighi, A., Shafipour, V., Bagheri-Nesami, M., Gholipour Baradari, A., & Yazdani Charati, J. (2017). The impact of oral care on oral health status and prevention of ventilator-associated pneumonia in critically ill patients. *Australian Critical Care, 30*(2), 69-73. doi:10.1016/j.aucc.2016.07.002

Hall, S. K., Robinson, P., & Green, A. (2000). Could salivary phenylalanine concentrations replace blood concentrations? *Annals of Clinical Biochemistry, 37*(Pt. 2), 222-223. doi:10.1258/0004563001899050

Harthoorn, L. F. (2008). Salivary α-amylase: A measure associated with satiety and subsequent food intake in humans. *International Dairy Journal, 18*(8), 879-883.

Hawkins, R. J. (1999). Functional status and untreated dental caries among nursing home residents aged 65 and over. *Special Care in Dentistry, 19*(4), 158-163.

Hector, M. P., & Linden, R. W. (1987). The possible role of periodontal mechanoreceptors in the control of parotid secretion in man. *Quarterly Journal of Experimental Physiology and Cognate Medical Sciences, 72*(3), 285-301.

Helmick, C. G., Felson, D. T., Lawrence, R. C., Gabriel, S., Hirsch, R., Kwoh, C. K., ... National Arthritis Data Workgroup. (2008). Estimates of the prevalence of arthritis and other rheumatic conditions in the United States: Part l. *Arthritis and Rheumatology, 58*(1), 15-25. doi:10.1002/art.23177.

Henson, B. S., Inglehart, M. R., Eisbruch, A., & Ship, J. A. (2001). Preserved salivary output and xerostomia-related quality of life in head and neck cancer patients receiving parotid-sparing radiotherapy. *Oral Oncology, 37*(1), 84-93. doi:10.1016/S1368-8375(00)00063-4

Hiiemae, K. M., Thexton, A. J., & Crompton, A. W. (1978). Intra-oral food transport: The fundamental mechanism of feeding. In D. S. Carlson & J. A. McNamara (Eds.), *Muscle Adaptation in the Craniofacial Region* (pp. 181-208). Ann Arbor, MI: University of Michigan.

Hillier, B., Wilson, C., Chamberlain, D., & King, L. (2013). Preventing ventilator-associated pneumonia through oral care, product selection, and application method: A literature review. *AACN Advanced Critical Care, 24*(1), 38-58. doi:10.1097/NCI.0b013e31827df8ad

Hiraba, H., Yamaoka, M., Fukano, M., Fujiwara, T., & Ueda, K. (2008). Increased secretion of salivary glands produced by facial vibrotactile stimulation. *Somatosensory and Motor Research, 25*(4), 222-229. doi:10.1080/08990220802611649

Ho, A., Affoo, R., Rogus-Pulia, N., Nicosia, M., Inamoto, Y., Saitoh, E., ... Fels, S. (2017). Inferring the effects of saliva on liquid bolus flow using computer simulation. *Computers in Biology and Medicine, 89*, 304-313. doi:10.1016/j.compbiomed.2017.07.014

Hoebler, C., Karinthi, A., Devaux, M. F., Guillon, F., Gallant, D. J., Bouchet, B., ... Barry, J. L. (1998). Physical and chemical transformations of cereal food during oral digestion in human subjects. *British Journal of Nutrition, 80*(5), 429-436. doi:10/1017/S0007114598001494

Hoek, G. H., Brand, H. S., Veerman, E. C., & Amerongen, A. V. (2002). Toothbrushing affects the protein composition of whole saliva. *European Journal of Oral Sciences, 110*(6), 480-481. doi:10.1034/j.1600-0722.2002.21370.x

Horner, J., Alberts, M. J., Dawson, D. V., & Cook, G. M. (1994). Swallowing in Alzheimer's disease. *Alzheimer Disease and Associated Disorders, 8*(3), 177-189.

Hughes, C. V., Baum, B. J., Fox, P. C., Marmary, Y., Yeh, C.-K., & Sonies, B. C. (1987). Oral-pharyngeal dysphasia: A common sequela of salivary gland dysfunction. *Dysphagia, 1*(4), 173-177. doi:10.1007/BF02406913

Humbert, I. A., McLaren, D. G., Kosmatka, K., Fitzgerald, M., Johnson, S., Porcaro, E., ... Robbins, J. (2010). Early deficits in cortical control of swallowing in Alzheimer's disease. *Journal of Alzheimer's Disease, 19*(4), 1185-1197. doi:10.3233/JAD-2010-1316

Humbert, I. A., McLaren, D. G., Malandraki, G., Johnson, S. C., & Robbins, J. (2011). Swallowing intentional off-state in aging and Alzheimer's disease: Preliminary study. *Journal of Alzheimer's Disease, 26*(2), 347-354. doi:10.3233/JAD-2011-110380

Humphrey, S. P., & Williamson, R. T. (2001). A review of saliva: Normal composition, flow, and function. *Journal of Prosthetic Dentistry, 85*(2), 162-169. doi:10.1067/mpr.2001.113778

Hutchings, J., & Lillford, P. (1988). The perception of food texture: The philosophy of the breakdown path. *Journal of Texture Studies, 19*(2), 103-115. doi: 10.1111/j.1745-4603.1988.tb00928.x

Hutchins, K., Karras, G., Erwin, J., & Sullivan, K. L. (2009). Ventilator-associated pneumonia and oral care: A successful quality improvement project. *American Journal of Infection Control, 37*(7), 590-597. doi:10.1016/j.ajic.2008.12.007

Jager, D. H. J., Bots, C. P., Forouzanfar, T., & Brand, H. S. (2018). Clinical oral dryness score: Evaluation of a new screening method for oral dryness. *Odontology, 106*(4), 439-444. doi:10.1007/s10266-018-0339-4

Jean, A. (1984). Control of the central swallowing program by inputs from the peripheral receptors. A review. *Journal of the Autonomic Nervous System, 10*(3-4), 225-233. doi:10.1016/0165-1838(84)90017-1

Kaneoka, A., Pisegna, J. M., Miloro, K. V., Lo, M., Saito, H., Riquelme, L. F., … Langmore, S. E. (2015). Prevention of healthcare-associated pneumonia with oral care in individuals without mechanical ventilation: A systematic review and meta-analysis of randomized controlled trials. *Infection Control & Hospital Epidemiology, 36*(8), 899-906. doi:10.1017/ice.2015.77

Kapila, Y. V., Dodds, W. J., Helm, J. F., & Hogan, W. J. (1984). Relationship between swallow rate and salivary flow. *Digestive Diseases and Sciences, 29*(6), 528-533. doi:10.1007/BF01296273

Kassan, S. S., & Moutsopoulos, H. M. (2004). Clinical manifestations and early diagnosis of Sjögren syndrome. *Archives of Internal Medicine, 164*(12), 1275-1284. doi:10.1001/archinte.164.12.1275

Kaya, H., Turan, Y., Tunal, Y., Aydın, G., Yüce, N., Gürbüz, Ş., & Tosun, K. (2017). Effects of oral care with glutamine in preventing ventilator-associated pneumonia in neurosurgical intensive care unit patients. *Applied Nursing Research, 33*, 10-14. doi:10.1016/j.apnr.2016.10.006

Kolenbrander, P. E., Palmer, R. J., Periasamy, S., & Jakubovics, N. S. (2010). Oral multispecies biofilm development and the key role of cell-cell distance. *Nature Reviews Microbiology, 8*(7), 471-480. doi:10.1038/nrmicro2381

Kuten, A., Ben-Aryeh, H., Berdicevsky, I., Ore, L., Szargel, R., Gutman, D., & Robinson, E. (1986). Oral side effects of head and neck irradiation: Correlation between clinical manifestations and laboratory data. *International Journal of Radiation Oncology • Biology • Physics, 12*(3), 401-405. doi:10.1016/0360-3016(86)90358-5

LaCroix, A. Z., Lipson, S., Miles, T. P., & White, L. (1989). Prospective study of pneumonia hospitalizations and mortality of U.S. older people: The role of chronic conditions, health behaviors, and nutritional status. *Public Health Reports, 104*(4), 350-360.

Lagerlöf, F., & Dawes, C. (1984). The volume of saliva in the mouth before and after swallowing, Journal of Dental Research, 63(5), 618-621. doi:10.1177/00220345840630050201

Lal, P., Nautiyal, V., Verma, M., Yadav, R., Maria Das, K. J., & Kumar, S. (2018). Objective and subjective assessment of xerostomia in patients of locally advanced head-and-neck cancers treated by intensity-modulated radiotherapy. *Journal of Cancer Research and Therapeutics, 14*(6), 1196-1201. doi:10.4103/jcrt.JCRT_200_17

Langmore, S. E., Terpenning, M. S., Schork, A., Chen, Y., Murray, J. T., Lopatin, D., & Loesche, W. J. (1998). Predictors of aspiration pneumonia: How important is dysphagia? *Dysphagia, 13*(2), 69-81. doi:10.1007/PL00009559

Lear, C. S., Catz, J., Grossman, R. C., Flanagan, J. B., & Moorrees, C. F. (1965). Measurement of lateral muscle forces on the dental arches. *Archives of Oral Biology, 10*(4), 669-690. doi:10.1016/0003-9969(65)90013-0

Li, Y., Taylor, J. M., Ten Haken, R. K., & Eisbruch, A. (2007). The impact of dose on parotid salivary recovery in head and neck cancer patients treated with radiation therapy. *International Journal of Radiation Oncology • Biology • Physics, 67*(3), 660-669. doi:10.1016/j.ijrobp.2006.09.021

Liedberg, B., & Owall, B. (1991). Masticatory ability in experimentally induced xerostomia. *Dysphagia, 6*(4), 211-213. doi:10.1007/BF02493529

Ligtenberg, A. J., Brand, H. S., Bots, C. P., & Nieuw Amerongen, A. V. (2006). The effect of toothbrushing on secretion rate, pH and buffering capacity of saliva. *International Journal of Dental Hygiene, 4*(2), 104-105. doi:10.1111/j.1601-5037.2006.00170.x

Lim, R. J., Nik Nabil, W. N., Chan, S. Y., Wong, Y. F., Han, L. X., Gong, J. Y., … Xu, L. (2019). Effects of herbal medicine for xerostomia in head and neck cancer patients: An observational study in a tertiary cancer hospital. *Support Care in Cancer.* doi:10.1007/s00520-019-4646-2

Liu, C., Cao, Y., Lin, J., Ng, L., Needleman, I., Walsh, T., & Li, C. (2018). Oral care measures for preventing nursing home-acquired pneumonia. *Cochrane Databases Systematic Review, 9*, CD012416. doi:10.1002/14651858.CD012416.pub2

Logemann, J. A. (1995). Dysphagia: Evaluation and treatment. *Folia Phoniatrica et Logopaedica, 47*(3), 140-164. doi:10.1159/000266348

Logemann, J. A., Pauloski, B. R., Colangelo, L., Lazarus, C., Fujiu, M., & Kahrilas, P. J. (1995). Effects of a sour bolus on oropharyngeal swallowing measures in patients with neurogenic dysphagia. *Journal of Speech, Language, and Hearing Research, 38*(3), 556-563. doi:10.1002/hed.1037

Logemann, J. A., Smith, C. H., Pauloski, B. R., Rademaker, A. W., Lazarus, C. L., Colangelo, L. A., … Newman, L. A. (2001). Effects of xerostomia on perception and performance of swallow function. *Head and Neck, 23*(4), 317-321. doi:10.1002/hed.1037

Longti, L., & Zheng X. J. (2015). Can routine oral care with antiseptics prevent ventilator-associated pneumonia in patients receiving mechanical ventilation? An update meta-analysis from 17 randomized controlled trials. *International Journal of Clinical and Experimental Medicine, 8*(2), 1645-1657.

Marik, P. E. (2001). Aspiration pneumonitis and aspiration pneumonia. *New England Journal of Medicine, 344*(9), 665-671. doi:10.1056/NEJM200103013440908

Matsuo, K. P., & Jeffery, B. (2013). Oral phase preparation and propulsion: Anatomy, rheology, mastication, and transport. In R. Shaker (Ed.), *Principles of Deglutition* (pp. 117-131). New York, NY: Springer.

Micik, S., Besic, N., Johnson, N., Han, M., Hamlyn, S., & Ball, H. (2013). Reducing risk for ventilator associated pneumonia through nursing sensitive interventions. *Intensive Critical Care Nursing, 29*(5), 261-265. doi:10.1016/j.iccn.2013.04.005

Miller, A. J. (2013). Overview of deglutition and digestion. In R. Shaker (Ed.), *Principles of Deglutition* (pp. 3-51). New York, NY: Springer.

Munro, C. L., & Grap, M. J. (2004). Oral health and care in the intensive care unit: State of the science. *American Journal of Critical Care, 13*(1), 25-33; discussion 34.

Murakami, M., Wei, M. X., Ding, W., & Zhang, Q. D. (2009). Effects of Chinese herbs on salivary fluid secretion by isolated and perfused rat submandibular glands. *World Journal of Gastroenterology, 15*(31), 3908-3915. doi:10.3748/wjg.15.3908

Namasivayam, A. M., & Steele, C. M. (2015). Malnutrition and dysphagia in long-term care: A systematic review. *Journal of Nutrition in Gerontology and Geriatrics, 34*(1), 1-21. doi:10.1080/21551197.2014.1002656

Navazesh, M., Christensen, C., & Brightman, V. (1992). Clinical criteria for the diagnosis of salivary gland hypofunction. *Journal of Dental Research, 71*(7), 1363-1369. doi:10.1177/00220345920710070301

Navazesh, M., & Ship, I. I. (1983). Xerostomia: Diagnosis and treatment. *American Journal of Otolaryngology, 4*(4), 283-292. doi:10.1016/S0196-0709(83)80072-6

Nederkoorn, C., Smulders, F., & Jansen, A. (1999). Recording of swallowing events using electromyography as a non-invasive measurement of salivation. *Appetite, 33*(3), 361-369. doi:10.1006/appe.1999.0268

Nik Nabil, W. N., Lim, R. J., Chan, S. Y., Lai, N. M., & Liew, A. C. (2018). A systematic review on Chinese herbal treatment for radiotherapy-induced xerostomia in head and neck cancer patients. *Complementary Therapies in Clinical Practice, 30*, 6-13. doi:10.1016/j.ctcp.2017.10.004

Osailan, S. M., Pramanik, R., Shirlaw, P., Proctor, G. B., & Challacombe, S. J. (2012). Clinical assessment of oral dryness: development of a scoring system related to salivary flow and mucosal wetness. *Oral Surgery, Oral Medicine, Oral Patholology and Oral Radiology, 114*(5), 597-603. doi:10.1016/j.oooo.2012.05.009

Padilha, D. M., Hugo, F. N., Hilgert, J. B., & Dal Moro, R. G. (2007). Hand function and oral hygiene in older institutionalized Brazilians. *Journal of the American Geriatrics Society, 55*(9), 1333-1338. doi:10.1111/j.1532-5415.2007.01278.x

Pai, S., Ghezzi, E. M., & Ship, J. A. (2001). Development of a visual analogue scale questionnaire for subjective assessment of salivary dysfunction. *Oral Surgery, Oral Medicine, Oral Patholology and Oral Radiology, 91*(3), 311-316. doi:10.1067/moe.2001.111551

Papas, A., Singh, M., Harrington, D., Rodríguez, S., Ortblad, K., de Jager, M., & Nunn, M. (2006). Stimulation of salivary flow with a powered toothbrush in a xerostomic population. *Special Care in Dentistry, 26*(6), 241-246. doi:10.1111/j.1754-4505.2006.tb01661.x

Park, B., Noh, H., & Choi, D. J. (2018). Herbal medicine for xerostomia in cancer patients: A systematic review of randomized controlled trials. *Integrative Cancer Therapies, 17*(2), 179-191. doi:10.1177/1534735417728336

Pedersen, A. M., Bardow, A., Jensen, S. B., & Nauntofte, B. (2002). Saliva and gastrointestinal functions of taste, mastication, swallowing and digestion. *Oral Diseases, 8*(3), 117-129. doi:10.1034/j.1601-0825.2002.02851.x

Petersen, P. E. & World Health Organization Oral Health Programme. (2003). The World Oral Health Report 2003: Continuous improvement of oral health in the 21st century—The approach of the WHO Global Oral Health Programme/Poul Erik Petersen. World Health Organization. Retrieved from http://www.who.int/iris/handle/10665/68506d

Peyron, M., Gierczynski, I., Hartmann, C., Loret, C., Dardevet, D., Martin, N., & Woda, A. (2011). Role of physical bolus properties as sensory inputs in the trigger of swallowing. *PLoS One, 6*(6), e21167. doi:10.1371/journal.pone.0021167

Poisson, P., Laffond, T., Campos, S., Dupuis, V., & Bourdel-Marchasson, I. (2016). Relationships between oral health, dysphagia and undernutrition in hospitalised elderly patients. *Gerodontology, 33*(2), 161-168. doi:10.1111/ger.12123

Preza, D., Olsen, I., Willumsen, T., Grinde, B., & Paster, B. J. (2009). Diversity and site-specificity of the oral microflora in the elderly. *European Journal of Clinical Microbiology & Infectious Diseases, 28*(9), 1033-1040. doi:10.1007/s10096-009-0743-3

Priefer, B. A., & Robbins, J. (1997). Eating changes in mild-stage Alzheimer's disease: A pilot study. *Dysphagia, 12*(4), 212-221. doi:10.1007/PL00009539

Prinz, J. F., & Lucas, P. W. (1995). Swallow thresholds in human mastication. *Archives in Oral Biology, 40*(5), 401-403. doi:10.1016/0003-9969(94)00185-E

Prinz, J. F., & Lucas, P. W. (1997). An optimization model for mastication and swallowing in mammals. *Proceedings of Royal Society B: Biological Sciences, 264*(1389), 1715-1721. doi:10.1098/rspb.1997.0238

Raynal, B. D. E., Hardingham, T. E., Sheehan, J. K., & Thornton, D. J. (2003). Calcium-dependent protein Interactions in MUC5B provide reversible cross-links in salivary mucus. *Journal of Biological Chemistry, 278*, 27803-27810. doi:10.1074/jbc.M304632200

Rhodus, N. L., & Bereuter, J. (2000). Clinical evaluation of a commercially available oral moisturizer in relieving signs and symptoms of xerostomia in postirradiation head and neck cancer patients and patients with Sjogren's syndrome. *Journal of Otolaryngology, 29*(1), 28-34.

Rhodus, N. L., Colby, S., Moller, K., & Bereuter, J. (1995). Quantitative assessment of dysphagia in patients with primary and secondary Sjögren's syndrome. *Oral Surgery, Oral Medicine, Oral Patholology, and Oral Radiology, 79*(3), 305-310.

Rhodus, N. L., Moller, K., Colby, S., & Bereuter, J. (1995). Dysphagia in patients with three different etiologies of salivary gland dysfunction. *Ear Nose and Throat Journal, 74*(1), 39-42, 45-38.

Richards, T., Hurley, T., Grove, L., Harrington, K., Carpenter, G., Proctor, G., & Nutting, C. (2017). The effect of parotid gland-sparing intensity-modulated radiotherapy on salivary composition, flow rate xerostomia measures. *Oral Diseases, 23*(7), 990-1000. doi:10.1111/odi.12686.

Rogus-Pulia, N. M., Gangnon, R., Kind, A., Connor, N. P., & Asthana, S. (2018). A pilot study of perceived mouth dryness, perceived swallowing effort, and saliva substitute effects in healthy adults across the age range. *Dysphagia, 33*(2), 200-205. doi:10.1007/s00455-017-9846-7

Rogus-Pulia, N. M., Larson, C., Mittal, B. B., Pierce, M., Zecker, S., Kennelty, K., … Connor, N. P. (2016). Effects of change in tongue pressure and salivary flow rate on swallow efficiency following chemoradiation treatment for head and neck cancer. *Dysphagia, 31*(5), 687-696. doi:10.1007/s00455-016-9733-7

Rogus-Pulia, N. M., & Logemann, J. A. (2011). Effects of reduced saliva production on swallowing in patients with Sjögren's syndrome. *Dysphagia, 26*(3), 295-303. doi:10.1007/s00455-010-9311-3

Rosenhek, M., Macpherson, L. M., & Dawes, C. (1993). The effects of chewing-gum stick size and duration of chewing on salivary flow rate and sucrose and bicarbonate concentrations. *Archives of Oral Biology, 38*(10), 885-891. doi:10.1016/0003-9969(93)90098-7

Rudney, J. D., Ji, Z., & Larson, C. J. (1995). The prediction of saliva swallowing frequency in humans from estimates of salivary flow rate and the volume of saliva swallowed. *Archives of Oral Biology, 40*(6), 507-512. doi:10.1016/0003-9969(95)00004-9

Running, C. A. (2018). Oral sensations and secretions. *Physiology and Behavior, 193*(Pt. B), 234-237. doi:10.1016/j.physbeh.2018.04.011

Rydholm, M., & Strang, P. (1999). Acupuncture for patients in hospital-based home care suffering from xerostomia. *Journal of Palliative Care, 15*(4), 20-23. doi:10.1177/082585979901500404

Scannapieco, F. A., Amin, S., Salme, M., & Tezal, M. (2017). Factors associated with utilization of dental services in a long-term care facility: A descriptive cross-sectional study. *Special Care in Dentistry, 37*(2), 78-84. doi:10.1111/scd.12208

Scannapieco, F. A., Torres, G., & Levine, M. J. (1993). Salivary alpha-amylase: Role in dental plaque and caries formation. *Critical Reviews in Oral Biology & Medicine, 4*(3-4), 301-307. doi:10.1177/10454411930040030701

Scott, J. (1977). A morphometric study of age changes in the histology of the ducts of human submandibular salivary glands. *Archives in Oral Biology, 22*(4), 243-249. doi:10.1016/0003-9969(77)90109-1

Scott, J., Flower, E. A., & Burns, J. (1987). A quantitative study of histological changes in the human parotid gland occurring with adult age. *Journal of Oral Pathology, 16*(10), 505-510. doi:10.1111/j.1600-0714.1987.tb00681.x

Ship, J. A., DeCarli, C., Friedland, R. P., & Baum, B. J. (1990). Diminished submandibular salivary flow in dementia of the Alzheimer type. *Journal of Gerontology, 45*(2), M61-M66. doi:10.1093/geronj/45.2.M61

Ship, J. A., & Puckett, S. A. (1994). Longitudinal study on oral health in subjects with Alzheimer's disease. *Journal of the American Geriatrics Society, 42*(1), 57-63.

Siegel, R. L., Miller, K. D., & Jemal, A. (2017). Cancer statistics, 2017. *CA: A Cancer Journal for Clinicians, 67*(1), 7-30. doi:10.3322/caac.21387

Skrinjar, I., Vucicevic Boras, V., Bakale, I., Andabak Rogulj, A., Brailo, V., Vidovic Juras, D., … Vrdoljak, D. V. (2015). Comparison between three different saliva substitutes in patients with hyposalivation. *Clinical Oral Investigations, 19*(3), 753-757. doi:10.1007/s00784-015-1405-8

Sreebny, L., & Schwartz, S. (1997). A reference to drugs and dry mouth. *Gerodontology, 14*(1), 33-47. doi:10.1111/j.1741-2358.1997.00033.x

Sreebny, L., & Vissink, A. (2010). *Dry mouth, the malevolent symptom: A clinical guide.* Iowa City, IA: Wiley-Blackwell.

Sreebny, L. M. (2000). Saliva in health and disease: An appraisal and update. *International Dental Journal, 50*(3), 140-161. doi:10.1111/j.1875-595X.2000.tb00554.x

Steele, C. M., & Miller, A. J. (2010). Sensory input pathways and mechanisms in swallowing: A review. *Dysphagia, 25*(4), 323-333. doi:10.1007/s00455-010-9301-5

Strietzel, F. P., Lafaurie, G. I., Mendoza, G. R., Alajbeg, I., Pejda, S., Vuletić, L., … Konttinen, Y. T. (2011). Efficacy and safety of an intraoral electrostimulation device for xerostomia relief: A multicenter, randomized trial. *Arthritis and Rheumatology, 63*(1), 180-190. doi:10.1002/art.27766

Suh, M-K., Kim, H., & Na, D. L. (2009). Dysphagia in patients with dementia: Alzheimer versus vascular. *Alzheimer Disease and Associated Disorders, 23*(2), 178-184. doi:10.1097/WAD.0b013e318192a539

Syrjänen, S. M., & Syrjänen, K. J. (1984). Inflammatory cell infiltrate in labial salivary glands of patients with rheumatoid arthritis with special emphasis on tissue mast cells. *Scandinavian Journal of Dental Research, 92*(6), 557-563. doi:10.1111/j.1600-0722.1984.tb01297.x

Tanaka, J., Ogawa, M., Hojo, H., Kawashima, Y., Mabuchi, Y., Hata, K., … Mishima, K. (2018). Generation of orthotopically functional salivary gland from embryonic stem cells. *Nature Communications, 9*(1), 4216. doi:10.1038/s41467-018-06469-7

Thexton, A. J. (1992). Mastication and swallowing: An overview. *British Dental Journal, 173*(6), 197-206. doi:10.1038/sj.bdj.4808002

Thomson, W. M., Chalmers, J. M., Spencer, A. J., & Williams, S. M. (1999). The Xerostomia Inventory: A multi-item approach to measuring dry mouth. *Community Dental Health, 16*(1), 12-17.

van der Bilt, A., Engelen, L., Pereira, L. J., van der Glas, H. W., & Abbink, J. H. (2006). Oral physiology and mastication. *Physiology and Behavior, 89*(1), 22-27. doi:10.1016/j.physbeh.2006.01.025

Vijay, A., Inui, T., Dodds, M., Proctor, G., Carpenter, G. (2015). Factors that influence the extensional rheological property of saliva. *PLoS ONE, 10*(8), e0135792. doi:10.1371/journal. pone.0135792

Volicer, L., Seltzer, B., Rheaume, Y., Karner, J., Glennon, M., Riley, M. E., & Crino, P. (1989). Eating difficulties in patients with probable dementia of the Alzheimer type. *Journal of Geriatric Psychiatry and Neurology, 2*(4), 188-195.

Wada, H., Nakajoh, K., Satoh-Nakagawa, T., Suzuki, T., Ohrui, T., Arai, H., & Sasaki, H. (2001). Risk factors of aspiration pneumonia in Alzheimer's disease patients. *Gerontology, 47*(5), 271-276. doi:52811

Wang, H., Zhou, M., Brand, J., & Huang, L. (2007). Inflammation activates the interferon signaling pathways in taste bud cells. *Journal of Neuroscience, 27*(40), 10703-10713. doi:10.1523/JNEUROSCI.3102-07.2007

Watanabe, S., & Dawes, C. (1988). The effects of different foods and concentrations of citric acid on the flow rate of whole saliva in man. *Archives of Oral Biology, 33*(1), 1-5. doi:10.1016/0003-9969(88)90089-1

Wei, H., & Yongming, Z. (2009). Function of traditional Chinese medicine in cancer radiotherapy and its prospect. *World Science and Technology, 11*(5), 742-746. doi:10.1016/S1876-3553(10)60035-X

Whelan, K. (2001). Inadequate fluid intakes in dysphagic acute stroke. *Clinical Nutrition, 20*(5), 423-428. doi:10.1054/clnu.2001.0467

Whelton, H. (2004). Introduction: The anatomy and physiology of salivary glands. In C. Dawes, W. M. Edgar, & D. M. O'Mullane (Eds.), *Saliva and oral health* (pp. 1-13). London, United Kingdom: British Dental Association.

Wiener, R. C., Wu, B., Crout, R., Wiener, M., Plassman, B., Kao, E., & McNeil, D. (2010). Hyposalivation and xerostomia in dentate older adults. *Journal of the American Dental Association, 141*(3), 279-284. doi:10.14219/jada. archive.2010.0161

Wolff, M., & Kleinberg, I. (1998). Oral mucosal wetness in hypo- and normosalivators. *Archives of Oral Biology, 43*(6), 455-462. doi:10.1016/S0003-9969(98)00022-3

Wong, H. (2013). Oral complications and management strategies for patients undergoing cancer therapy. *The Scientific World Journal, 4*(4), 581795. doi:10.1155/2014/581795

Yeh, C. K., Johnson, D. A., Dodds, M. W., Sakai, S., Rugh, J. D., & Hatch, J. P. (2000). Association of salivary flow rates with maximal bite force. *Journal of Dental Research, 79*(8), 1560-1565. doi:10.1177/00220345000790080601

Voice Disorders and Xerostomia

Kristine Tanner, PhD, CCC-SLP

Xerostomia and voice disorders coexist in many patient populations. Underlying disease processes may explain many of these cases, necessitating comprehensive, interdisciplinary care.

Practitioners in subspecialties should ensure that appropriate referrals are made to maximize patient outcomes and overall quality of life. Recent research has increased the understanding of the unified airway, resulting in the development of novel treatments to manage and possibly prevent dryness-related voice disorders. This chapter includes an overview of hydration in the airway, vocal health, clinical voice care, at-risk populations, and emerging treatments.

Voice and Hydration

Hydration is essential for healthy voice function (Finkelhor, Titze, & Durham, 1988; Sivasankar & Fisher, 2002). Symptoms of vocal fold dehydration can include oropharyngeal and laryngeal dryness, hoarseness, cough, viscous mucus, vocal strain, and fatigue, to name a few (Solomon, Glaze, Arnold, & van Mersbergen, 2003; Verdolini-Marston, Sandage, & Titze, 1994; Verdolini et al., 2002). Xerostomia, pharyngeal, and laryngeal dryness symptoms are highly correlated, presumably due to influences such as the close proximity of anatomic structures, shared somatosensory mechanisms, and overlapping endogenous and environmental risk factors for dryness (Heller et al., 2014; Ruiz Allec et al., 2011; Sivasankar, Erickson, Schneider, & Hawes, 2008). People who are at risk for vocal fold dehydration may make behavioral adjustments to compensate for these dryness symptoms. Over time, compensatory behavioral adjustments can cause chronic voice disorders, impairing everyday communication, psychosocial health, and overall quality of life (Merrill et al., 2013; Roy et al., 2004).

Historically, xerostomia was considered to be an ancillary, even unrelated, symptom to voice disorders in many clinical voice circles. Few practitioners, predominantly those working with head and neck cancer and autoimmune disease populations, documented the coexistence of xerostomia and voice problems (Doig, Whaley, Dick, Nuki, Williamson, & Buchanan, 1971; Hocevar-Boltezar,

Ginsberg, S. M. (Ed.).
Xerostomia: An Interdisciplinary Approach to Managing Dry Mouth (pp. 99-115).
© 2020 Taylor & Francis Group.

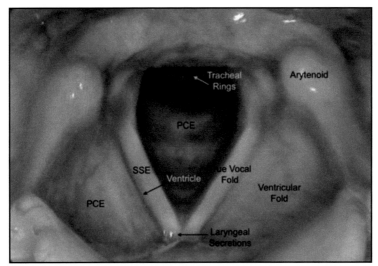

Figure 7-1. A superior view of a normal female larynx, including labeled true vocal folds, ventricular folds, arytenoid cartilages, tracheal rings, and areas of pseudostratified columnar epithelium and stratified squamous epithelium. Also labeled are the laryngeal entrance to the laryngeal ventricle and the collection of laryngeal secretions at the anterior portion of the vocal folds. (PCE = pseudostratified columnar epithelium; SSE = stratified squamous epithelium.)

Zargi, & Strojan, 2009); the relationships among xerostomia, and other health conditions, and voice disorders remained poorly understood. Limited referrals among practitioners serving these populations was an indication of the lack of understanding regarding xerostomia and other voice-related conditions. However, recent theoretical and clinical advances regarding conditions of the nose, mouth, throat, and lungs, or the *unified airway*, have begun to determine the physiologic underpinnings for inter-relationships among upper and lower respiratory health, injury, and treatment (Krouse et al., 2007). Thus, working within the framework of the unified airway, this chapter addresses fundamental principles of vocal health, the relationship between xerostomia and voice disorders, and emerging treatments for these conditions.

HYDRATION OF THE RESPIRATORY TRACT

The upper respiratory system is composed broadly of the nose, mouth, pharynx, and larynx, whereas the lower respiratory system includes the trachea, bronchi, bronchioles, and alveoli. The biomechanics of respiration incorporate active and passive forces involving the chest wall, pulmonary system, respiratory musculature, and nervous system control (Hoit & Weismer, 2016). Ciliated pseudostratified columnar epithelial cells line the majority of the respiratory tract from the lower bronchioles to the nares. These epithelial cells also line the larynx, with the exception of the stratified, nonciliated squamous epithelium that covers the true vocal folds. Similarly, the oral cavity transitions to stratified squamous cell, nonciliated epithelium. One of the significant characteristics of the pseudostratified columnar epithelium is the presence of goblet cells that secrete mucus. There are also glands that secrete mucus, including laryngeal glands that lubricate the vocal folds and salivary glands that moisten the mouth (Kacmarek, Stoller, & Heuer, 2017). Figure 7-1 displays the anatomic landmarks of the larynx, including epithelial cell types and significant structures.

The mucus in the respiratory tract serves several functions. It forms a matrix that is important to epithelial cell protection, immune response, and airway clearance. Mucus traps potential irritants and pollutants that may then be expelled during cough or clearance via ciliary beating

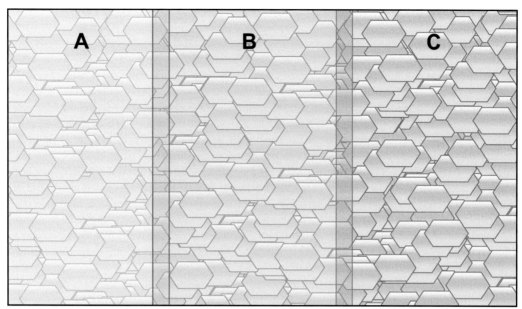

Figure 7-2. A simplified three-dimensional illustration of the gel layer that covers the surface of the vocal folds. (A) The most superficial view from the direction of the airway lumen; the mucus matrix (pale yellow layer) travels from the lungs toward the mouth and interacts with the sol layer that covers epithelial cells. (B) A deeper view of the gel layer, including only the sol layer (clear layer) and epithelial cells. (C) The unorganized hexagonal surface cells of the stratified squamous vocal fold epithelium (blue layer). Collectively, these layers filter, hydrate, and protect the deeper layers of the vocal fold epithelium and facilitate healthy voice function.

(Levendoski, Leydon, & Thibeault, 2014; Yeates, 1991). During routine upper respiratory illness, additional mucus secretions assist with the immune system response and the eventual return of airway health. A water, or *sol*, layer covers the airway surface epithelial cells, influencing the viscosity, spinnability, and mobility of the mucus blanket above (Widdicombe, 1997). Together, the mucus and sol layers form a gel that lubricates the vocal folds and facilitates healthy voice function. Likewise, hydration of the airway surface epithelial cells interacts with the depth of the sol layer and the overall health of the respiratory tract (Fisher, Ligon, Sobecks, & Roxe, 2001). Airway surface hydration, including the vocal folds, occurs via both internal, or systemic, and external, or surface-level, environmental mechanisms (Sivasankar et al., 2008). Figure 7-2 is a simplified illustration of the mucus-water blanket on the surface epithelial cells of the true vocal fold stratified squamous epithelium.

SYSTEMIC VERSUS SURFACE HYDRATION

To meet the growing need for voice disorder treatment and prevention in at-risk populations, an increasing body of research addresses relationships between dryness, epithelial health, and voice function. Broadly, this research involves systemic and surface-level dehydration mechanisms in ex vivo and human models (Hemler, Wieneke, & Dejonckere, 1997; Hocevar-Boltezar et al., 2009; Sivasankar, Nofziger, & Blazer-Yost, 2008; Sivasankar & Erickson, 2009; Witt et al., 2009). Systemic hydration is the process whereby adequate extracellular fluid levels are maintained in order to provide necessary nutrients to the vital organs and tissues via cellular transport mechanisms. The renal system is the main regulator of systemic hydration levels, supplied primarily by the oral intake of fluids. Systemic hydration has been the topic of significant research in areas of human physiology and sports medicine (American College of Sports Medicine et al., 2007; Montain, 2008). The majority of this work has focused on possible mechanisms for maintaining adequate systemic hydration levels to maximize performance and prevent dehydration.

Systemic Hydration Alterations

Voice practitioners have long suggested that individuals must be conscientious in their fluid intake in order to maximize voice quality. These recommendations have been particularly prevalent among singers, actors, and professional voice users (Fisher et al., 2001; Van Wyk, Cloete, Hattingh, van der Linde, & Geertsema, 2017); however, evidence for an association between voice disorders and changes in systemic hydration is still limited. In order to appreciate the relative risks for voice changes associated with systemic hydration levels, a review of hydration regulation is warranted. Generally, extracellular fluid levels are maintained quite precisely, and changes in the range of 200 to 300 mL result in immediate alterations in thirst and urine output (Hartley & Thibeault, 2014; Popkin, D'Anci, & Rosenberg, 2010). Although mild *hypohydration* (i.e., less than normal total body water) is fairly common, particularly in young athletes and older adults, significant alterations are associated with serious health conditions such as hypernatremia and cerebral edema. Similarly, *clinical dehydration* is defined as an inadequate ratio of fluid intake vs output, occurring most frequently with acute gastrointestinal illness or extreme exercise. Alternatively, *hyperhydration* may occur in situations involving excessive water intake, such as health conditions involving dysregulated thirst and cases of water torture (Armstrong, 2007).

Internally, the vocal folds require adequate fluid within and between tissues for efficient vocal fold vibration. Fluid regulation occurs via ionic transport mechanisms, ensuring that the viscosity of the fluid in the vocal fold layers is not too high. Evidence from vibratory biomechanics indicates that as the viscosity of the fluid within the vocal folds increases, the pulmonary pressure required to produce voice also increases. *Phonation threshold pressure* (PTP) is the primary outcome measure in hydration-related voice research and is defined as the minimum amount of subglottic pressure required to initiate and sustain vocal fold vibration (Titze, 1994). PTP is modestly correlated with vocal effort and laryngeal dryness. Therefore, decreases in vocal fold viscosity produce desirable reductions in PTP and corresponding improvements in voice quality, but, collectively, the results from studies involving the manipulation of systemic hydration alone to influence voice function have been mixed (Solomon & DiMattia, 2000; Solomon et al., 2003).

Surface Tissue Hydration Alterations

More recently, vocal fold surface tissue hydration has received greater attention in the literature. Vocal fold surface fluid is continuous with the gel layer that covers the airway epithelium and serves lubricating and hydrating functions. The vocal fold epithelium is porous and responsive to the osmotic gradient and active transport mechanisms (Sivasankar et al., 2008). It has been theorized that fluid may move bidirectionally across the vocal fold epithelial surface for purposes of cellular health. When the gel layer becomes too viscous on the vocal fold surface, a corresponding increase in pulmonary pressure is needed for voice production. Similar to the internal effects of fluid viscosity, increases in fluid viscosity on the vocal fold surface result in the collection of thick, tacky mucus; increased vocal effort; and decreased voice efficiency.

The majority of research involving vocal fold surface fluid involves the combination of both systemic and surface hydration variables. These studies include the manipulation of the oral intake of fluids; environmental humidity; and the ingestion of drugs such as antihistamines, mucolytics, or caffeine (Verdolini-Marston, Titze, & Druker, 1990; Verdolini-Marston et al., 1994; Verdolini et al., 2002). Collectively, the results from this body of work indicate that perturbations in vocal fold surface fluid influence voice function, but additional research and improved measures are needed to determine the clinical relevance of factors that affect laryngeal dryness and associated voice disorders (Alves, Krüger, Pillay, van Lierde, & van der Linde, 2019; Leydon, Sivasankar, Falciglia, Atkins, & Fisher, 2009; Sivasankar & Leydon, 2010).

Hydration and Vocal Health

Voice practitioners have included hydration in their clinical recommendations to promote vocal health for decades (Stemple, Roy, & Klaben, 2014). Hydration practices also have a long-standing history in vocal pedagogy to optimize voice use in singing and theater. Professional voice users have been likened to vocal athletes, and hydration is often deeply entrenched in an individual's performance regimen. As such, it is important to consider individuals' investments in their own vocal health practices before recommending any significant changes. For example, performers might report improved voice immediately after drinking water even though the fluid bypasses the larynx completely during swallowing. Those who work with performers should also review these practices for any that might have potentially adverse effects, such as the consumption of refluxogenic items in an individual at risk for acid reflux. Steam inhalation, lozenges, teas, herbal supplements, alkaline water, sports drinks, and beverages that purport to improve oropharyngeal and laryngeal hydration are commonplace; however, it is noteworthy that little is known about the sensory effects the use of such items might have in those who use them routinely. Just like any other motor learning routine, it is possible that these practices might have a sensorimotor, or even a placebo or psychomotor, effect that ultimately results in greater confidence and consequently improved performance in different populations. Furthermore, it has been established that xerostomia, throat dryness, and vocal effort are correlated (Tanner et al., 2013; Tanner, Nissen, et al., 2015; Tanner, Stevens, Berardi, Titze, & Sivasankar, 2016). These factors notwithstanding, it is essential that the voice practitioner evaluate critically each of these practices to determine their relative risk vs. benefit.

Overview of Clinical Voice Care

Clinical voice disorders encompass structural, functional, or neurologic diagnostic categories (Stemple et al., 2014). Another common diagnostic framework is organic (i.e., structural and neurologic) vs. functional (i.e., behavioral or muscle tension based; American Speech-Language-Hearing Association, n.d.). These categories are not mutually exclusive, and functional disorders routinely overlap with structural or neurologic disorders. Additionally, a variety of other health conditions may overlap with voice disorders and are considered during assessment and treatment planning. Structural disorders involve phonotraumatic, or presumably use-based, lesions on the vocal folds (e.g., vocal nodules and polyps), as well as other congenital and acquired growths, such as those related to human papilloma virus and laryngeal cancer. Neurologic voice disorders may be focal, such as vocal fold paralysis or spasmodic dysphonia, or may be related to another neurodegenerative condition such as Parkinson's disease. Functional disorders are those attributed to excess or dysregulated musculoskeletal tension in the laryngeal region; they are often referred to as *muscle tension dysphonia*, are very common, and can be quite severe despite having a normal vocal fold appearance. Although functional dysphonia is not organic in nature, it is typically highly responsive to behavioral voice therapy. Only extremely rarely are these disorders psychogenic in origin, requiring formal diagnosis by a mental health professional with corresponding expertise in voice disorders.

An interdisciplinary approach is essential for appropriate assessment and management of voice disorders. It is common for patients to present in voice clinics for voice evaluation when there is actually an underlying, undiagnosed health condition or disease process contributing in whole or part to the disorder. This is particularly true for conditions that affect multiple speech subsystems such as neurodegenerative disease processes, but this also occurs with other diseases, such as those involving autoimmune function. When patients present with xerostomia and voice disorders, they may not yet have been diagnosed with the underlying cause for these symptoms. Therefore, the interdisciplinary team must be watchful for signs and symptoms of conditions that are associated with xerostomia, such as certain autoimmune diseases, and make appropriate referrals. This continuity of care is also important to the differential diagnosis of voice disorders that might initially be categorized as functional (e.g., muscle tension dysphonia) or phonotraumatic (e.g., vocal nodules) when, in fact, xerostomia could be correlated with the laryngeal manifestation of another disease process (e.g., vocal fold inflammation or rheumatoid/bamboo nodules). Thus, the relationships among xerostomia, laryngeal dryness, respiratory symptoms, and voice problems must be thoroughly vetted.

Comprehensive voice assessment involves a laryngologist (i.e., an otolaryngology subspecialty with voice fellowship or extensive clinical voice training) and a speech-language pathologist with specific expertise in voice and upper airway disorders. Interdisciplinary assessment may take several forms, but, ideally, individuals are evaluated by the team together so that they can confer regarding the diagnosis, optimal treatment plan, and timeline for management and follow-up. Because voice patients are often seen as part of a tertiary, or subspecialty, care center, it is important to reach out to other appropriate team members. These team members may be from a variety of disciplines depending on the origin of the referral, the diagnosis, and treatment plan but most frequently include primary care, pulmonology, gastroenterology, neurology, cardiology, rheumatology, endocrinology, dental providers, voice teachers and coaches, otolaryngologists from other subspecialties (e.g., sinus), speech-language pathologists, and family members or care providers. This list of team members is far from comprehensive and is dynamic based on the nature of the voice disorder.

As the format or sequence of interdisciplinary assessment varies by patient preferences, individual practice patterns, insurance plans, and regional considerations, to name a few, it is essential that team members communicate in a timely manner with each other to reach a consensus on the best management plan. Generally, voice evaluation includes the following:

- Case history
- Review of symptoms
- Physical examination
- Clinician-based perceptual measures
- Patient-based perceptual measures
- Aerodynamic instrumental measures
- Acoustic instrumental measures
- Videolaryngostroboscopy

Importantly, patients must receive laryngeal imaging if a voice problem does not resolve within a 4-week period, or sooner if there is concern about an urgent health matter such as vocal fold hemorrhage or cancer (Stachler et al., 2018). If behavioral voice therapy is recommended for a structural, functional, or neurologic voice disorder, the average course of treatment often ranges from six to eight visits over a 2-month period (American Speech-Language-Hearing Association, n.d.). The treating speech-language pathologist should communicate with the laryngologist or referring physician during therapy if the patient does not improve; additionally, any follow-up visits or referrals should be completed or adjusted as needed to optimize patient outcomes. Voice assessment and management should follow current best practice patterns and evidence-based techniques. The American Academy of Otolaryngology, the American Laryngological Association, and the American-Speech-Language-Hearing Association comprise oversight boards and coordinate practice guidelines for clinical voice care.

At-Risk Populations

Currently, over 107 million Americans are at risk for dryness-related conditions of the unified airway, including xerostomia and laryngeal dehydration. Populations at greatest risk include adults and children with asthma, allergies, sleep apnea, and certain autoimmune diseases and those living in dry climates (Doig et al., 1971; Erickson & Sivasankar, 2010; Hamdan, Sabra, Rifai, Tabri, &

Hussari, 2008; King, Dube, & Homa, 2013; Merrill, Anderson, & Sloan, 2011; Stewart, Ferguson, & Fromer, 2010; Trangsrud, Whitaker, & Small, 2002). Additionally, the growing number of medications causing dryness of the unified airway, including dehydration of the vocal folds, is staggering (Christensen, 2012). Therefore, the number of people with or at risk for voice disorders associated with unified airway dryness is rising. Other populations at risk for dryness-related voice disorders include individuals with vocal fatigue, benign vocal fold lesions, hypersensitive airways, professional voice users, and those treated for head and neck cancers.

Autoimmune Disease

In clinical voice settings, autoimmune diseases are one of the most frequently seen conditions that are associated with both xerostomia and dehydration-related voice disorders (Stemple et al., 2014). The growing body of research and related clinical reports on this topic indicates that often these patients have not been identified as having an underlying disease process at the time of the initial evaluation. Signs and symptoms of unified airway dryness are identified, and then the patient is referred for additional testing and evaluation by the appropriate specialist. In general, this is the standard of care for laryngologists caring for voice patients. Additionally, speech-language pathologists with specialty expertise in voice disorders are familiar with autoimmune-related xerostomia and dryness symptoms and work with the interdisciplinary team and referring physician to coordinate appropriate medical follow-up (Ruiz Allec et al., 2011).

Sjögren's syndrome is an autoimmune disease that is characterized classically by symptoms of xerostomia, dry eyes, dry throat, and voice problems (Newton et al., 2012; Ogut et al., 2005). The criteria for diagnosing Sjögren's syndrome have changed quite recently, but it is generally determined by the combination of standardized physical examinations, blood work, and cheek or lip biopsy (Brito-Zerón et al., 2016; Freeman, Sheehan, Thorpe, & Rutka, 2005). This disease process may be primary or secondary to another autoimmune condition. When the disease takes a more severe form, the dryness effects are systemic. Additional symptoms include neuropathy and increased risk for the development of lymphoma. Recent epidemiological research indicates that Sjögren's syndrome has a high prevalence of current dryness-associated voice disorders (approximately 60%), and the communication-related disease burden is high (Pierce et al., 2015; Tanner, Pierce, et al., 2015). Overlapping issues with speech production, dentition, and voice use are common. Due to the complexity of this condition, the importance of interdisciplinary management of this condition cannot be overstated.

Other autoimmune conditions frequently associated with xerostomia and voice disorders include rheumatoid arthritis, systemic lupus erythematosus, scleroderma, and other mixed connective tissue diseases (Iacovou, Vlastarakos, & Nikolopoulos, 2014; Immerman & Sulica, 2007; Roy et al., 2016). These disease processes can have unpredictable effects on voice and speech, including inflammation, vocal fold lesions, and peripheral neuropathy. Diabetes is another condition that falls loosely under the umbrella of autoimmune-related voice disorders. In general, inflammatory conditions of the larynx seem to overlap with autoimmune processes including associated oropharyngeal and laryngeal dryness symptoms and voice disorders. Sarcoidosis is one such condition that can result in severe, debilitating, and precancerous lesions on the vocal folds. Furthermore, the demand for additional research on inflammatory processes in the unified airway, including those affecting voice, is significant (Hanshew, Jetté, Rosen, & Thibeault, 2017). Endocrinology is an important addition to the interdisciplinary team when addressing the complexity and evolving theoretical frameworks regarding how best to care for patients with autoimmune diseases.

Hypersensitive Airway

Asthma, paradoxical vocal cord dysfunction, chronic cough, sleep apnea, allergies, and chronic upper respiratory conditions, such as rhinitis and sinusitis, also include associated risks of xerostomia and dryness-related voice disorders. Conditions that are characterized by restricted or obstructed nasal breathing put patients at risk for xerostomia, adverse impact on dental health, and voice problems. Mouth breathing for durations as short as 15 minutes causes significant increases in PTP and vocal effort (Sivasankar & Erickson-Levendoski, 2012; Sivasankar & Fisher, 2002, 2003). Additionally, treatments to manage underlying conditions, such as continuous positive airway pressure treatment for sleep apnea and the adverse effects of combination inhaled corticosteroids in asthma, may actually lead to worsening of oropharyngeal and laryngeal symptoms (Erickson & Sivasankar, 2010; Sahrawat, Robb, Kirk, & Beckert, 2014; Sivasankar & Blazer-Yost, 2009). Viscous laryngeal mucus secretions associated with the immune response to hypersensitive airway conditions also make the vocal fold surface stickier, increasing the amount of respiratory pressure and effort required for voice production. Other conditions with compromised respiratory systems, such as airway stenosis, cystic fibrosis, and tracheostomy with or without ventilator dependence, are associated with risk of dryness due to impaired mucociliary clearance, more rapid breathing, and thicker mucus. These symptoms may be exacerbated in particularly dry climates.

Head and Neck Cancer

Individuals with head and neck cancer are a diverse population with a range of presentations and symptoms. The risks for xerostomia and associated voice disorders are dependent largely on the type and location of the cancer as well as the treatments received. For example, the prevalence of oropharyngeal cancers associated with human papilloma virus is one of the fastest rising in the United States (Chaturvedi et al., 2011); this form of cancer is particularly aggressive, attacking the stratified squamous epithelium in the mouth and the vocal folds. Treatment can leave patients with xerostomia and laryngeal dryness, in addition to further serious complications such as difficulty swallowing. Other cancers, such as those affecting the salivary or lymph glands, are associated with dryness, as are certain treatment protocols such as those involving radiation. Patient education and speech-language pathology services before surgical management are key during the coordination of care for these individuals (Ward & van As-Brooks, 2014).

Vocal Health Concerns

It is important to consider that the current understanding of precise physiologic mechanisms responsible for dryness-related voice disorders is very limited. This is due in part to measurement tool limitations. Some clinical inferences may be made by applying principles of the unified airway to speech and voice. For example, it is known that PTP increases with vocal nodules because the subglottal pressure must overcome greater vocal fold mass and medial compression. Speech utterances are also generally shorter in those with nodules due to the loss of air through an hourglass-shaped glottis during vibration. This loss of air during phonation requires the speaker to breathe more frequently. Similarly, patients with presbylaryngis have a spindle-shaped glottal configuration during phonation, resulting in shorter utterances and more frequent breathing. It is quite possible that more frequent respiration during speech might provoke xerostomia and dryness-related voice problems, potentially even perpetuating the voice disorder unless treated (Sivasankar & Erickson-Levendoski, 2012). In a similar vein, very little is understood regarding the relationship between sensory information and vocal performance with respect to dryness symptoms. Significant work is needed to develop quantitative, clinically relevant measures to determine the effects of xerostomia and pharyngeal and laryngeal dryness in specific structural, functional, and neurologic voice disorders.

EMERGING TREATMENTS

Voice treatment corresponds to respective structural, functional, and neurologic disorder diagnoses. Ideally, interdisciplinary evaluation, including diagnostic therapy and therapeutic probes, inform treatment planning and overall prognosis. A number of evidence-based resources are available to guide the management of voice disorder management (American Speech-Language-Hearing Association, n.d.; Van Stan, Roy, Awan, Stemple, & Hillman, 2015). Behavioral voice therapy is recommended for patients who are stimulable or have a likelihood of improvement with therapeutic management. Speech-language pathologists with voice expertise use a variety of evidence-based treatment techniques to facilitate voice improvement. This typically involves in-person or telehealth sessions with regular home practice to promote generalization and maintenance. Vocal hygiene, including hydration recommendations, and patient counseling related to voice problems are an indirect approach that provides an essential, but not stand-alone, component of treatment. Direct approaches include specific vocal exercises and practice regimens that are aimed at stimulating and maintaining improved voice production. It is important to note that, despite underlying health conditions that might exist, many patients with xerostomia and voice disorders respond well to voice therapy in the hands of skilled clinicians using evidence-based techniques.

Topical hydration is a gold standard for preventing and treating dryness of the skin, eyes, nose, and mouth (Aukema & Fokkens, 2004; Badami & McKellar, 2012; Reeves, Molloy, Pohl, & McElvaney, 2012). Oral lubricants and moisture-promoting products are common recommendations for individuals with xerostomia. Nasal irrigation using saline-based sinus rinses improves upper respiratory health and nasal breathing. Treating the vocal folds topically is more complex due to anatomic position and airway protection mechanisms that prevent food and liquid from contacting the vocal folds. These challenges notwithstanding, topical treatments are important because systemic hydration is insufficient to prevent vocal fold dehydration in at-risk populations.

Environmental Humidity

Research indicates that increasing the ambient humidity of a room produces corresponding improvements in voice quality (Erickson-Levendoski, Sundarrajan, & Sivasankar, 2014; Finkelhor et al., 1988; Verdolini-Marston et al., 2002). Breathing dry air by mouth for as little as 15 minutes results in quantifiable changes in vocal effort (Sivasankar & Fisher, 2002, 2003). Nasal breathing has been shown to reverse these changes in individuals with normal voices as well as those who experience vocal fatigue. Mouth breathing also leads to xerostomia; therefore, preventing situations in which an individual must rely on mouth breathing in dry environments can manage both symptoms. Optimizing room humidity levels is a fairly low-maintenance, inexpensive method for addressing oropharyngeal and laryngeal dryness. The most significant challenges seem to be reaching a high enough humidity level and the lack of humidification portability within and between environments. Dryness-provoking short-term illnesses, such as upper respiratory infections, may be mitigated by humidifying the room environment and applying adhesive nasal strips at night, but chronic xerostomia and dryness-related voice disorders pose greater challenges for long-term management. Central humidifiers in the home and monitoring with a calibrated hygrometer can be useful in maximizing exposure to high humidity environments.

There are a variety of humidifier styles and a broad range of price points. The two main subtypes are fan and ultrasonic. Fan-style humidifiers use a spinning disk or fan mechanism to distribute water from the tank into the surrounding air. These humidifiers are often loud at the fan source and require filters to reduce mineral output; this can also be accomplished by using distilled water to fill the tank. The fan-style humidifiers require that filters be changed consistently and that the tank and internal components be thoroughly cleaned on a regular, usually weekly, basis. The other type of humidifier is ultrasonic, which is generally much quieter and produces greater water output. Ultrasonic humidifiers do not require filters; however, it is important to clean the tank regularly per manufacturer instructions to prevent the growth of bacteria. Although the output is greater than fan humidifiers, the water particles are often larger and may not travel as far in the air. These factors vary by the size, type, and placement of the humidifier in the environment.

Another method for increasing environmental humidity is with the use of vaporizers. These devices also vary in size and price range. Vaporizers heat the water in the tank until it boils and thus convert particles to a steam that is distributed into the environment. Because they are steam driven, most vaporizers are of the warm mist variety. Those vaporizers that offer warm and cool settings typically combine a traditional warm mist vaporizer with a cool mist humidifier mechanism that may be set by the user. Again, vaporizers must be cleaned regularly, including filter replacement. Notably, any solute added to the vaporizer, such as salt, is not actually distributed into the atmosphere. Salt simply increases the electrical conductivity between the electrodes to facilitate efficient steam production. Eucalyptus or other additives may be delivered as a vapor or strong odor into the air in certain types of vaporizers. In summary, environmental humidification is a low-cost and effective way to treat dryness-related conditions of the oropharynx and larynx. It is possible that regular use may also have some preventive effect when used before entering a dry environment (e.g., airplane travel, stage performances, vigorous exercise).

Water Mist

More direct and portable approaches to hydrating the upper respiratory tract have been attempted to treat or prevent oropharyngeal and laryngeal dryness. These approaches include steam inhalation, facial steamers, and facial mist devices. Until recently, there was no research evidence to support the use of steam inhalation (Mahalingam & Boominathan, 2016). Traditionally, steam inhalation has been used to relieve symptoms of acute upper respiratory infection but was unlikely to produce any significant effect on voice function. Yet, facial steamers (i.e., portable vaporizers) and personal facial mist devices (i.e., portable ultrasonic humidifiers) have gained popularity in voice communities, particularly among performers and professional voice users. The most significant limitation to these personal steam or mist devices relates to water particle size. These devices are essentially miniature versions of humidifiers or vaporizers, which were designed to deliver water particles to environmental air and not directly to the respiratory tract. As such, the majority of particles are most likely deposited in the nose and mouth but are not small enough to travel to the level of the vocal folds. Table 7-1 provides a summary of particle sizes that are filtered by structures in the nose, mouth, throat, and lower airways. Additionally, caution is warranted when inhaling steam to prevent burns. Furthermore, if aerosolized water particles reach the vocal folds, a cough reflex is triggered; this reflex is used by pulmonary medicine practitioners to induce sputum and has been well documented. Thus, any water particles that might reach the larynx via these devices would trigger cough and counteract any potentially therapeutic effect. With that being said, the possible benefits of these devices in treating xerostomia alone, with possible sensory carryover to the larynx, merit further investigation.

Nebulized Saline

One promising new topical vocal fold hydration treatment is aerosolized (nebulized) saline. Saline is a natural hydration treatment routinely used for the nose and sinuses (Aukema & Fokkens, 2004). More recently, saline has been used to improve respiratory health in patients with pulmonary disease (Reeves et al., 2012). Ex vivo canine and porcine studies also confirm that vocal fold dehydration can be treated topically with liquid saline applications (Sivasankar et al., 2008; Witt et al., 2009; Witt, Taylor, Regner, & Jiang, 2011). Most recently, aerosolized isotonic saline (0.9% Na^+Cl^-) prophylactically offset the adverse effects of a desiccation challenge on PTP (Tanner et al., 2016). Figure 7-3 illustrates typical vocal fold closure in a young female at baseline, after a 15-minute desiccation challenge (oral breathing of dry air with < 1% relative humidity), and after 3 mL nebulized

Table 7-1. Particle Size Filtration for the Unified Airway During Inhalation

ANATOMIC LANDMARKS	PARTICLE SIZE FILTRATION

• Nose
  ○ Nares
  ○ Turbinates
  ○ Septum
  ○ Sinuses
  ○ Nasopharynx
  ○ Velopharyngeal port
	> 10 μm deposit in nasal cavity

• Mouth
  ○ Lips
  ○ Cheeks
  ○ Tongue
  ○ Dentition
  ○ Hard palate
  ○ Faucial pillars
  ○ Tonsils
  ○ Soft palate
  ○ Oropharynx
	> 15 μm deposit in oral cavity

• Throat
  ○ Tongue base
  ○ Epiglottis
  ○ Arytenoid cartilages
  ○ Aryepiglottic folds
  ○ Ventricular folds
  ○ True vocal folds
  ○ Pyriform sinuses
  ○ Laryngopharynx
	> 5 to 10 μm deposit in the laryngopharyngeal cavities

• Trachea • Main stem bronchi	> 5 to 10 μm deposit in this portion of the lower airway
• Bronchioles • Alveoli	< 1 to 5 μm reach this portion of the lower airway

Note: Particles larger than the respective filtration size are likely to deposit on the corresponding structures and not move further into the respiratory tract during inhalation (Elliott & Dunne, 2011).

isotonic saline administered via an ultrasonic nebulizer. Notably, vocal fold closure was poor after the desiccation challenge and returned to baseline after nebulized treatment. Therefore, a discussion of the potential effects of aerosolized saline to treat and prevent xerostomia and dryness-related voice disorders is warranted.

Figure 7-3. High-speed endoscopy of healthy vocal folds of a 26-year-old female at (A) baseline, (B) after a 15-minute oral breathing desiccation challenge, and (C) after nebulizing 3 mL isotonic saline (0.9% Na^+Cl^-) via an ultrasonic nebulizer. Note the poor vocal fold closure during the desiccation challenge and the improved closure after the nebulized treatment.

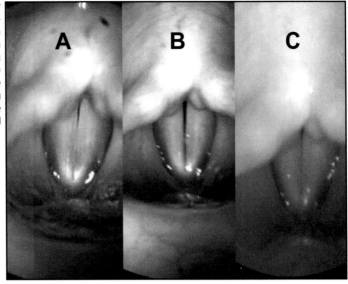

Nebulizers are devices that convert liquid into small particles that may be inhaled. Most nebulizers are produced for use in pulmonary medicine to treat conditions such as asthma or chronic obstructive pulmonary disease. Therefore, nebulizers are optimized to deliver particles to the lower airway and thus designed to produce particles less than 5 μm in size. Although the lower airway is the traditional target for nebulized treatments, many particles deposit in the oral cavity, pharynx, larynx, and trachea before reaching the lungs (Elliott & Dunne, 2011). Figure 7-4 is a photograph of dyed saline particles deposited in a silicone vocal tract model during simulated respiration for 3 minutes. Similarly, Figure 7-5 shows a comparison of air compressor (jet) vs ultrasonic nebulizers regarding saline particles deposited in the oropharynx, at or below the vocal folds, vs. lost to the atmosphere during 3 minutes of simulated respiration. This demonstrates why only a fraction of the drug delivered is considered therapeutic to the lower airway, but this apparent disadvantage might be exploited if particles could be delivered to the unified airway as a treatment for oropharyngeal and laryngeal dryness.

Many factors influence how particles are received in the unified airway. One must consider the mucus and water gel layer that lines the respiratory tract, the different types of epithelial cells, mucociliary clearance, glandular secretions, epithelial ionic transport mechanisms, and the airway's response to potential irritants. For example, if an individual inhales dust, mucus and salivary secretions increase and cough reflexes occur, ultimately trapping and expelling the majority of the irritant from the airway. During this sequence of events, the secretion of mucus and ionic transport responses send lubrication in the direction of the airway lumen. The additional secretions might produce a short-lived advantage for vocal fold vibration, but there is a net disadvantage to the airway. Therefore, any substance introduced to the airway for purposes of hydration should not adversely disturb airway homeostasis.

Early research in this area involved the use of a compressed air nebulizer to deliver three types of particles (liquid mannitol, sterile water, and Entertainer's Secret Throat Relief) to young, healthy females. Liquid mannitol was chosen due to its large particle size and potential to draw fluid into the airway lumen via the osmotic gradient. Entertainer's Secret Throat Relief is a glycerin-based product selected due to widespread use among performers; sterile water served as a control. The results indicated that the large-particle mannitol produced short-lived decreases in PTP in contrast to the other two liquids (Roy, Tanner, Gray, Blomgren, & Fisher, 2003). Subsequently, the effects of nebulized hypertonic saline (7% Na^+Cl^-), isotonic saline (0.9% Na^+Cl^-), and sterile water were examined in a double-blind, placebo-controlled study involving females with normal voices. Hypertonic saline

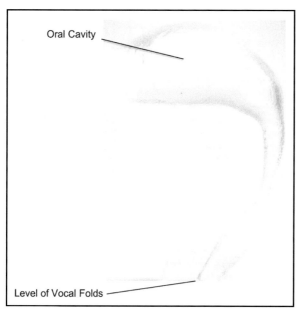

Oral Cavity

Level of Vocal Folds

Figure 7-4. Stained aerosolized saline oropharyngeal deposition in a three-dimensional silicone vocal tract model after simulated respiration. The silicone model was created from a three-dimensional print of the oropharynx in a neutral "ah" respiration posture. Vocal tract geometry was based on prior vocal tract magnetic resonance imaging research (Story, Titze, & Hoffman, 1996).

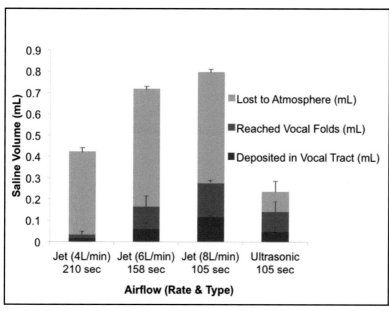

Figure 7-5. The proportion of saline particles that reach the level of the vocal folds vs. those lost to the vocal tract or atmosphere (mean and standard deviation for two trials each).

was selected to manipulate the osmotic gradient in the direction of the airway lumen, whereas isotonic saline was theorized to have a minimal effect on epithelial water flux due to its similarity to extracellular fluid in the human body. A 15-minute desiccation challenge (i.e., oral breathing of medical-grade dry air with less than 1% relative humidity) was completed immediately before nebulized treatment administration. The results showed that isotonic saline produced a short-lived reversal of the adverse effects of the desiccation challenge on PTP (Tanner, Roy, Merrill, & Elstad, 2007). Similar results were observed in a later study involving classically trained sopranos (Tanner et al., 2010).

Subsequently, nebulized isotonic saline was studied using a similar within-subjects design in adult male singers and nonsingers (Tanner et al., 2016) and in adult males and females with primary Sjögren's syndrome (Heller et al., 2014; Tanner et al., 2013). Then, in an 8-week longitudinal

Figure 7-6. PTP (cm H$_2$O) before and after 4 minutes of aerosolized isotonic saline (0.9% Na$^+$Cl$^-$) applied topically via an ultrasonic nebulizer (mean and standard deviation for five benchtop-mounted freshly excised porcine larynges). Isotonic saline was applied liberally via a spray bottle during fine dissection and upon mounting. Post-PTP values indicate improved voice function after nebulized saline administration despite traditional spray saline application immediately prior.

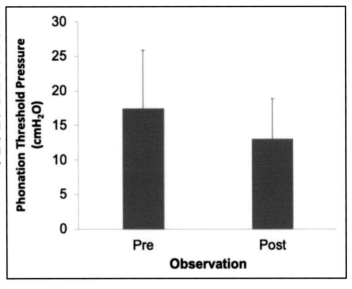

study using an ABAB experimentally controlled within-subjects design, adult females with primary Sjögren's syndrome demonstrated significant improvements in acoustic measures of voice function, as well as mouth dryness, throat dryness, and vocal effort during ultrasonic nebulized isotonic saline use at a 9-mL twice-daily dose (Tanner, Nissen, et al., 2015). High correlations among mouth dryness, throat dryness, and voice function were also demonstrated in these studies. Findings have also been replicated recently in public school teachers (Santana, Masson, & Araújo, 2017). Important next steps include dose-related parameters, the development of improved measurement tools, and the application of these treatments to other voice disorders. The results from recent pilot work displayed in Figure 7-6 indicate that ultrasonic nebulized isotonic saline might improve voice function even when the vocal folds are already lubricated. Ultimately, this body of work shows great promise in addressing coexisting xerostomia and dryness or dehydration-related voice disorders.

ACKNOWLEDGMENTS

Portions of the author's research cited in this chapter were supported by the David O. McKay School of Education, Brigham Young University and grant 1R01DC016269-01A1 from the National Institute on Deafness and Other Communication Disorders, National Institutes of Health. Special thanks are given to students working in the author's laboratory on research cited in this chapter, including collaborative efforts with the Department of Mechanical Engineering, Brigham Young University.

REFERENCES

Alves, M., Krüger, E., Pillay, B., van Lierde, K., & van der Linde, J. (2019). The effect of hydration on voice quality in adults: A systematic review. *Journal of Voice, 33*, 125. doi:10.1016/j.jvoice.2017.10.001

American College of Sports Medicine, Sawka, M. N., Burke, L. M., Eichner, E. R., Maughan, R. J., Montain, S. J., & Stachenfeld, N. S. (2007). American College of Sports Medicine position stand. Exercise and fluid replacement. *Medicine & Science in Sports & Exercise, 39*, 377-390. doi:10.1249/mss.0b013e31802ca597

American Speech-Language-Hearing Association. (n.d.). Voice disorders [Practice Portal]. Retrieved from https://www.asha.org/Practice-Portal/Clinical-Topics/Voice-Disorders/

Armstrong, L. E. (2007). Assessing hydration status: The elusive gold standard. *Journal of the American College of Nutrition, 26*, 575S-584S. doi:10.1080/07315724.2007.10719661

Aukema, A. A., & Fokkens, & W. J. (2004). Chronic rhinosinusitis: Management for optimal outcomes. *Treatments in Respiratory Medicine, 3*, 97-105. doi:10.2165/00151829-200403020-00004

Badami, K. G., & McKellar, M. (2012). Allogeneic serum eye drops: Time these became the norm? *British Journal of Ophthalmology, 96*, 1151-1152. doi:10.1136/bjophthalmol-2012-301668

Brito-Zerón, P., Theander, E., Baldini, C., Seror, R., Retamozo, S., Quartuccio, L., … Ramos-Casals, M. (2016). Early diagnosis of primary Sjögren's syndrome: EULAR-SS task force clinical recommendations. *Expert Review in Clinical Immunology, 12*, 137-156. doi:10.1586/1744666X.2016.1109449

Chaturvedi, A. K., Engels, E. A., Pfeiffer, R. M., Hernandez, B. Y., Xiao, W., Kim, E., … Gillison, M. L. (2011). Human papillomavirus and rising oropharyngeal cancer incidence in the United States. *Journal of Clinical Oncology, 29*, 4294-4301. doi:10.1200/JCO.2011.36.4596

Christensen, G. J. (2012). Common prescriptions associated with xerostomia. *Clinicians Report.* Retrieved from https://www.cliniciansreport.org/uploads/files/55/Meds%20Cause%20Xerostomia.pdf

Doig, J. A., Whaley, K., Dick, W. C., Nuki, G., Williamson, J., & Buchanan, W. W. (1971). Otolaryngological aspects of Sjögren's syndrome. *British Medical Journal, 4*, 460-463.

Elliott, D., & Dunne, P. (2011). *Guide to aerosol delivery device for physicians, nurses, pharmacists, and other health care professionals* (pp. 1-64). Irving, TX: American Association for Respiratory Care.

Erickson, E., & Sivasankar, M. (2010). Evidence for adverse phonatory change following an inhaled combination treatment. *Journal of Speech, Language, and Hearing Research, 53*, 75-83. doi:10.1044/1092-4388(2009/09-0024)

Erickson-Levendoski, E., Sundarrajan, A., & Sivasankar, M. P. (2014). Reducing the negative vocal effects of superficial laryngeal dehydration with humidification. *Annals of Otology, Rhinology, and Laryngology, 123*, 475-481.

Finkelhor, B. K., Titze, I. R., & Durham, P. L. (1988). The effect of viscosity changes in the vocal folds on the range of oscillation. *Journal of Voice, 1*, 320-325. doi:10.1016/S0892-1997(88)80005-5

Fisher, K. V., Ligon, J., Sobecks, J. L., & Roxe, D. M. (2001). Phonatory effects of body fluid removal. *Journal of Speech, Language, and Hearing Research, 44*, 354-367. doi:10.1044/1092-4388(2001/029)

Freeman, S. R., Sheehan, P. Z., Thorpe, M. A., & Rutka, J. A. (2005). Ear, nose, and throat manifestations of Sjögren's syndrome: Retrospective review of an interdisciplinary clinic. *Journal of Otolaryngology, 34*, 20-24. doi:10.2310/7070.2005.00020

Hamdan, A. L., Sabra, O., Rifai, H., Tabri, D., & Hussari, A. (2008). Vocal changes in patients using nasal continuous positive airway pressure. *Journal of Voice, 22*, 603-606. doi:10.1016/j.jvoice.2006.12.005

Hanshew, A. S., Jetté, M. E., Rosen, S. P., & Thibeault, S. L. (2017). Integrating the microbiota of the respiratory tract with the unified airway model. *Respiratory Medicine, 126*, 68-74. doi:10.1016/j.rmed.2017.03.019

Hartley, N. A., & Thibeault, S. L. (2014). Systemic hydration: Relating science to clinical practice in vocal health. *Journal of Voice, 28*, 652. doi:10.1016/j.jvoice.2014.01.007

Heller, A., Tanner, K., Roy, N., Nissen, S. L., Merrill, R. M., Miller, K. L., … Kendall, K. (2014). Voice, speech, and laryngeal features of primary Sjögren's syndrome. *Annals of Otology, Rhinology, and Laryngology, 123*, 778-785. doi:10.1177/0003489414538762

Hocevar-Boltezar, I., Zargi, M., & Strojan, P. (2009). Risk factors for voice quality after radiotherapy for early glottic cancer. *Radiotherapy and Oncology, 93*, 524-529. doi:10.1016/j.radonc.2009.09.014

Hoit, J. D., & Weismer, G. (2016). *Foundations of speech and hearing: Anatomy and physiology.* San Diego, CA: Plural Publishing.

Iacovou, E., Vlastarakos, P. V., & Nikolopoulos, T. P. (2014). Laryngeal involvement in connective tissue disorders. Is it important for patient management? *Indian Journal of Otolaryngology, Head and Neck Surgery, 66*, 22-29.

Immerman, S., & Sulica, L. (2007). Bamboo nodes. *Otolaryngology-Head and Neck Surgery, 137*, 162-163. doi:10.1016/j.otohns.2006.12.027

Kacmarek, R. M., Stoller, J. K., & Heuer, A. J. (2017). *Egan's fundamentals of respiratory care* (11th ed.). St. Louis, MO: Elsevier.

King, B. A., Dube, S. R., & Homa, D. M. (2013). Smoke-free rules and secondhand smoke exposure in homes and vehicles among US adults, 2009-2010. *Preventing Chronic Disease, 10*, E79. doi:10.5888/pcd10.120218

Krouse, J. H., Brown, R. W., Fineman, S. M., Han, J. K., Heller, A. J., Joe, S., … Veling, M. C. (2007). Asthma and the unified airway. *Otolaryngology-Head and Neck Surgery, 136*, S75-S106. doi:10.1016/j.otohns.2007.02.019

Levendoski, E. E., Leydon, C., & Thibeault, S. L. (2014). Vocal fold epithelial barrier in health and injury: A research review. *Journal of Speech, Language, and Hearing Research, 57*, 1679-1691. doi:10.1044/2014_JSLHR-S-13-0283

Leydon, C., Sivasankar, M., Falciglia, D. L., Atkins, C., & Fisher, K. V. (2009). Vocal fold surface hydration: A review. *Journal of Voice, 23*, 658-665. doi:10.1016/j.jvoice.2008.03.010

Mahalingam, S., & Boominathan, P. (2016). Effects of steam inhalation on voice quality-related acoustic measures. *The Laryngoscope, 126*, 2305-2309.

Merrill, R. M., Anderson, A. E., & Sloan, A. (2011). Quality of life indicators according to voice disorders and voice-related conditions. *The Laryngoscope, 121*, 2004-2010. doi:10.1002/lary.21895

Merrill, R. M., Tanner, K., Merrill, J. G., McCord, M. D., Beardsley, M. M., & Steele, B. A. (2013). Voice symptoms and voice-related quality of life in college students. *Annals of Otology, Rhinology, and Laryngology, 122*, 511-519. doi:10.1177/000348941312200806

Montain, S. J. (2008). Hydration recommendations for sport 2008. *Current Sports Medicine Reports, 7*, 187-192. doi:10.1249/JSR.0b013e31817f005f.

Newton, J. L., Frith, J., Powell, D., Hackett, K., Wilton, K., Bowman, S., … Ng, W. F. (2012). Autonomic symptoms are common and are associated with overall symptom burden and disease activity in primary Sjögren's syndrome. *Annals of the Rheumatic Diseases, 71*, 1973-1979. doi:10.1136/annrheumdis-2011-201009

Ogut, F., Midilli, R., Oder, G., Engin, E. Z., Karci, B., & Kabasakal, Y. (2005). Laryngeal findings and voice quality in Sjögren's syndrome. *Aurus Nasus Larynx, 32*, 375-380. doi:10.1016/j.anl.2005.05.016

Pierce, J. L., Tanner, K., Merrill, R. M., Miller, K. L., Ambati, B. K., Kendall, K. A., & Roy, N. (2015). Voice disorders in Sjögren's syndrome: Prevalence and related risk factors. *The Laryngoscope, 125*, 1385-1392.

Popkin, B. M., D'Anci, K. E., & Rosenberg, I. H. (2010). Water, hydration, and health. *Nutrition Reviews, 68*, 439-458. doi:0.1111/j.1753-4887.2010.00304

Reeves, E. P., Molloy, K., Pohl, K., & McElvaney, N. G. (2012). Hypertonic saline in treatment of pulmonary disease in cystic fibrosis. *Scientific World Journal, 2012*, 465230. doi:10.1100/2012/465230

Roy, N., Merrill, R. M., Thibeault, S., Parsa, R. A., Gray, S. D., & Smith, E. M. (2004). Prevalence of voice disorders in teachers and the general population. *Journal of Speech, Language, and Hearing Research, 47*, 281-293. doi:10.1044/1092-4388(2004/023)

Roy, N., Tanner, K., Gray, S., Blomgren, M., & Fisher, K. (2003). An evaluation of the effects of three laryngeal lubricants on phonation threshold pressure (PTP). *Journal of Voice, 17*, 331-342.

Roy, N., Tanner, K., Merrill, R. M., Wright, C., Miller, K. L., & Kendall, K. A. (2016). Descriptive epidemiology of voice disorders in rheumatoid arthritis: Prevalence, risk factors, and quality of life burden. *Journal of Voice, 30*, 74-87.

Ruiz Allec, L. D., Lopez, X. H., Porras, J. B., Ramos, R. V., Valle, J. C., & Garcia, A. I. (2011). Alterations in voice, speech and swallowing in patients with Sjögren's syndrome. *Acta Otorrinolaringológica Española, 62*, 255-264. doi:10.1016/j.otorri.2010.12.011

Sahrawat, R., Robb, M. P., Kirk, R., & Beckert, L. (2014). Effects of inhaled corticosteroids on voice production in healthy adults. *Logopedics, Phoniatrics, Vocology, 39*, 108-116. doi:10.3109/14015439.2013.777110

Santana, E. R., Masson, M. L. V., & Araújo, T. M. (2017). The effect of surface hydration on teachers' voice quality: An intervention study. *Journal of Voice, 31*, 383.e5-383.e11. doi:10.1016/j.jvoice.2016.08.019

Sivasankar, M. P., & Blazer-Yost, B. (2009). Effects of long-acting beta adrenergic agonists on vocal fold ion transport. *The Laryngoscope, 119*, 602-607.

Sivasankar, M., & Erickson, E. (2009). Short-duration accelerated breathing challenges affect phonation. *The Laryngoscope, 119*, 1658-1663. doi:10.1002/lary.20530

Sivasankar, M., Erickson, E., Schneider, S., & Hawes, A. (2008). Phonatory effects of oral breathing: Preliminary evidence for impaired compensation to airway dehydration in individuals with vocal fatigue. *Journal of Speech, Language, and Hearing Research, 51*, 1494-1506. doi:10.1044/1092-4388(2008/07-0181)

Sivasankar, M. P., & Erickson-Levendoski, E. (2012). Influence of obligatory mouth breathing, during realistic activities, on voice measures. *Journal of Voice, 26*, 813. doi:10.1016/j.voice.2012.03.007

Sivasankar M., & Fisher K. V. (2002). Oral breathing increases Pth and vocal effort by superficial drying of vocal fold mucosa. *Journal of Voice, 16*, 172-181. doi:10.1016/S0892-1997(02)00087-5

Sivasankar, M., & Fisher, K. V. (2003). Oral breathing challenge in participants with vocal attrition. *Journal of Speech, Language, and Hearing Research, 46*, 1416–1427. doi:10.1044/1092-4388(2003/110)

Sivasankar, M., & Leydon, C. (2010). The role of hydration in vocal fold physiology. *Current Opinion in Otolaryngology & Head and Neck Surgery, 18*, 171-175. doi:10.1097/MOO.0b013e3283393784

Sivasankar, M., Nofziger, C., & Blazer-Yost, B. (2008). Cyclic adenosine monophosphate regulation of ion transport in porcine vocal fold mucosa. *The Laryngoscope, 118*, 1511-1517. doi:10.1097/MLG.0b013e3181772d63

Solomon, N. P., & DiMattia, M. S. (2000). Effects of a vocally fatiguing task and systemic hydration on phonation threshold pressure. *Journal of Voice, 14*, 341-362. doi:10.1016/S0892-1997(00)80080-6

Solomon, N. P., Glaze, L. E., Arnold, R. R., & van Mersbergen, M. (2003). Effects of a vocally fatiguing task and systemic hydration on men's voices. *Journal of Voice, 17*, 31-46. doi:10.1016/S0892-1997(03)00029-8

Stachler, R. J., Francis, D. O., Schwartz, S. R., Damask, C. C., Digoy G. P., Krousem H. J., … Nnacheta, L. C. (2018). Clinical practice guideline: Hoarseness (dysphonia) (update). *Otolaryngology—Head and Neck Surgery, 158*, S1-S42. doi:10.1177/0194599817751030

Stemple, J. C., Roy, N., & Klaben, B. K. (2014). *Clinical voice pathology: Theory and management* (5th ed.). San Diego, CA: Plural Publishing.

Stewart, M., Ferguson, B. J., & Fromer, L. (2010). Epidemiology and burden of nasal congestion. *International Journal of General Medicine, 3,* 37-45.

Story, B. H., Titze, I. R., & Hoffman, E. A. (1996). Vocal tract area functions from magnetic resonance imaging. *Journal of the Acoustical Society of America, 100,* 537-554.

Tanner, K., Fujiki, R. B., Dromey, C., Merrill, R. M., Robb, W., Kendall, K. A., … Sivasankar, M. P. (2016). Laryngeal desiccation challenge and nebulized isotonic saline in healthy male singers and nonsingers: Effects on acoustic, aerodynamic, and self-perceived effort and dryness measures. *Journal of Voice, 30,* 670-676.

Tanner, K., Nissen, S. L., Merrill, R. M., Miner, A., Channell, R. W., Miller, K. L., … Roy, N. (2015). Nebulized isotonic saline improves voice production in Sjögren's syndrome. *The Laryngoscope, 125,* 2333-2340.

Tanner, K., Pierce, J. L., Merrill, R. M., Miller, K. L., Kendall, K. A., & Roy, N. (2015). The quality of life burden associated with voice disorders in Sjögren's syndrome. *Annals of Otology, Rhinology, and Laryngology, 124,* 721-727.

Tanner, K., Roy, N., Merrill, R. M., & Elstad, M. (2007). The effects of three nebulized osmotic agents in the dry larynx. *Journal of Speech, Language, and Hearing Research, 50,* 635-646.

Tanner, K., Roy, N., Merrill, R. M., Elstad, M., Kendall, K., Miller, K., … Houtz, D. (2013). Comparing nebulized water versus saline after laryngeal desiccation challenge in Sjögren's syndrome. *The Laryngoscope, 123,* 2787-2792

Tanner, K., Roy, N., Merrill, R. M., Muntz, F., Houtz, D., Sauder, C., … Wright-Costa, J. (2010). Nebulized isotonic saline versus water following a laryngeal desiccation challenge in classically-trained sopranos. *Journal of Speech, Language, and Hearing Research, 53,* 1555-1566.

Tanner, K., Stevens, M. E., Berardi, M. L., Titze, I. R., & Sivasankar, M. P. (2016, July 7). A translational prophylactic model for environmental laryngeal perturbation. Paper presented at the Modeling Laryngeal Biology Bi-Annual Symposium, Madison, WI.

Titze, I. R. (1994). *Principle of voice production.* Englewood Cliffs, NJ: Prentice-Hall.

Trangsrud, A. J., Whitaker, A. L., & Small, R. E. (2002). Intranasal corticosteroids for allergic rhinitis. *Pharmacotherapy, 22,* 1458-1467. doi:10.1592/phco.22.16.1458.33692

Van Stan, J. H., Roy, N., Awan, S., Stemple, J., & Hillman, R. E. (2015). A taxonomy of voice therapy. *American Journal of Speech-Language Pathology, 24,* 101-125. doi:10.1044/2015_AJSLP-14-0030

Van Wyk, L., Cloete, M., Hattingh, D., van der Linde, J., & Geertsema, S. (2017). The effect of hydration on the voice quality of future professional vocal performers. *Journal of Voice, 31,* 111. doi:10.1016/j.jvoice.2016.01.002

Verdolini-Marston, K., Min, Y., Titze, I. R., Lemke, J., Brown, K., van Mersbergen, M., … Fisher, K. (2002). Biological mechanisms underlying voice changes due to dehydration. *Journal of Speech, Language, and Hearing Research, 45,* 268-281. doi:10.1044/1092-4388(2002/021)

Verdolini-Marston, K., Sandage, M., & Titze, I. R. (1994). Effect of hydration treatments on laryngeal nodules and polyps and related voice measures. *Journal of Voice, 8,* 30-47. doi:10.1016/S0892-1997(05)80317-0

Verdolini-Marston, K., Titze, I. R., & Druker, D. G. (1990). Changes in phonation threshold pressure with induced conditions of hydration. *Journal of Voice, 4,* 142-151. doi:10.1016/S0892-1997(05)80139-0

Ward, E. C., & van As-Brooks, C. J. (2014). *Head and neck cancer: Treatment, rehabilitation, and outcomes* (2nd ed.). San Diego, CA: Plural Publishing.

Widdicombe, J. (1997). Airway surface liquid: Concepts and Measurements. In D. F. Rogers & M. Lethem (Eds.), *Airway mucus: Basic mechanisms and clinical perspectives* (pp. 1-17). Basel, Switzerland: Birkhauser, Verlag.

Witt, R. E., Regner, M. F., Tao, C., Rieves, A. L., Zhuang, P., & Jiang, J. J. (2009). Effects of dehydration on phonation threshold flow in excised canine larynges. *Annals of Otology, Rhinology, and Laryngology, 118,* 154-159. doi:10.1177/000348940911800212

Witt, R. E., Taylor, L. N., Regner, M. F., & Jiang, J. J. (2011). Effects of surface dehydration on mucosal wave amplitude and frequency in excised canine larynges. *Otolaryngology—Head and Neck Surgery, 144,* 108-113. doi:10.1177/0194599810390893

Yeates, D. (1991). Mucus rheology. In J. B. West (Ed.), *The lung: Scientific foundations* (pp. 197-203). New York, NY: Raven.

8

Pharmacological Management of Xerostomia

Sharon Ingersoll, PharmD

Dry mouth is a common side effect for many chronic medications; yet, patients are often not aware of the potential for this adverse effect. Pharmacists are in a unique position to identify potential drug-related xerostomia, to consult with primary care providers on potential alternative medications, and to consult with health care professionals and patients regarding over-the-counter (OTC) and prescription treatment options. Drugs that are known to cause xerostomia are discussed in this chapter. The pharmacology associated with various treatment options is reviewed. The role of the pharmacist in managing xerostomia is discussed, and practical considerations for patients are provided.

Causative Agents (Drug-Induced Xerostomia)

Dry mouth, or xerostomia, is listed as an adverse event in over 500 marketed prescription drugs (Porter, Scully, & Hegarty, 2004) and is associated with an increased risk of dental caries, mucosal soreness, and, in more severe cases, malnourishment related to difficulty eating and swallowing. The top 200 drugs dispensed in the United States in 2016 represent 90% of the annual prescriptions filled (ClinCalc, 2018). Of these top 200 medications, 40% have xerostomia listed as a potential adverse drug reaction (ADR) and are included in Table 8-1 (Lexicomp, 2018). The drugs contained in Table 8-1 are sorted alphabetically by generic name to facilitate rapid lookup of commonly prescribed drugs that may cause xerostomia. Other studies estimate the percentage of commonly prescribed drugs in the United States (Sreebny & Schwartz, 1997) and Canada (Nguyen, MacEntee, Mintzes, & Perry, 2014) associated with dry mouth to be 61% to 63%.

A list of therapeutic subgroups (therapeutic drug classes) associated with these commonly prescribed drugs that are reported to cause xerostomia are provided in Table 8-2 (ClinCalc, 2018; Clinical Pharmacology, 2018; Lexicomp, 2018). The drugs contained in Table 8-2 are sorted by anatomic group and therapeutic subgroup to assist in searching for commonly prescribed drugs by drug class. The therapeutic subgroups align with the international World Health Organization (2018) therapeutic drug classification system, reflecting the organ system associated with each medication listed.

Ginsberg, S. M. (Ed.)
Xerostomia: An Interdisciplinary Approach to Managing Dry Mouth (pp. 117-165).
© 2020 Taylor & Francis Group.

Table 8-1. Commonly Dispensed Drugs Listing Xerostomia as a Potential Adverse Drug Reaction

DRUG NAME	ATC CLASSIFICATION	DRUG NAME	ATC CLASSIFICATION
Acetaminophen/ hydrocodone	N02	Clonazepam	N04
Albuterol	R01	Clonidine	C02
Albuterol/ipratropium	R01	Cyclobenzaprine	M03
Alprazolam	N05	Dexlansoprazole	A01
Amiodarone	C01	Dextroamphetamine/ amphetamine	N07
Amitriptyline	N06	Diazepam	N05
Amlodipine	C07	Diclofenac	M01
Amlodipine/benazepril	C07	Dicyclomine	A07
Aripiprazole	N05	Diltiazem	C07
Atenolol	C07	Donepezil	N06
Baclofen	M03	Dorzolamide/timolol	S01
Beclomethasone	R01	Doxazosin	C02
Benazepril	C09	Doxycycline	J01
Brimonidine	S01	Duloxetine	N06
Budesonide/ formoterol	R03	Enalapril	C09
Bupropion	N06	Escitalopram	N06
Calcium/cholecalciferol	A11	Esomeprazole	A02
Canagliflozin	A10	Famotidine	A02
Carbamazepine	N03	Fenofibrate	C10
Carbidopa/levodopa	N04	Fluconazole	J02
Carisoprodol	M03	Fluoxetine	N06
Carvedilol	C07	Fluticasone	R01
Celecoxib	M01	Fluticasone/salmeterol	R01
Cetirizine	R06	Gabapentin	N03
Ciprofloxacin	J01	Guanfacine	C02
Citalopram	N06	Hydrochlorothiazide/ lisinopril	C03

(continued)

Table 8-1 (continued). Commonly Dispensed Drugs Listing Xerostomia as a Potential Adverse Drug Reaction

DRUG NAME	ATC CLASSIFICATION	DRUG NAME	ATC CLASSIFICATION
Hydrochlorothiazide/ losartan	C03	Nortriptyline	N06
Hydrochlorothiazide/ triamterene	C03	Omeprazole	A02
		Ondansetron	A04
Hydrochlorothiazide/ valsartan	C03	Oxybutynin	G04
		Oxycodone	N02
Hydrocodone	N02	Pantoprazole sodium	A02
Hydroxyzine	N05	Paroxetine	N06
Ibuprofen	M01	Pregabalin	N03
Ipratropium	R03	Progesterone	G03
Isosorbide	C04	Promethazine	R06
Lamotrigine	N03	Quetiapine	N05
Lansoprazole	A02	Ramipril	C09
Levocetirizine	R06	Risperidone	N05
Liraglutide	A10	Ropinirole	N04
Lisdexamfetamine	N06	Sertraline	N06
Lisinopril	C09	Solifenacin	G04
Loratadine	R06	Sumatriptan	N02
Losartan	C09	Tamsulosin	G04
Lovastatin	C10	Terazosin	G04
Meclizine	A04	Testosterone	G03
Meloxicam	M01	Tiotropium	R03
Methylphenidate	N06	Tizanidine	M03
Metoprolol	C07	Topiramate	N03
Metronidazole	J01	Tramadol	N02
Mirtazapine	N06	Trazodone	N06
Mometasone	R03	Triamcinolone	R01
Morphine	N02	Valsartan	C09
Mupirocin	R01	Venlafaxine	N06
Naproxen	M01	Verapamil	C08
Nifedipine	C08	Zolpidem	N05
Nitroglycerin	C04		

Adapted from ClinCalc (2018), Clinical Pharmacology (2018), and Lexicomp Online (2018).

ATC = Anatomical Therapeutic Chemical classification code.

Table 8-2. Drug Classes Associated With Commonly Dispensed Drugs Listing Xerostomia as a Potential Adverse Drug Reaction

ATC LEVEL 1 ANATOMIC GROUP	ATC LEVEL 2 THERAPEUTIC SUBGROUP	ATC LEVEL 5 CHEMICAL SUBSTANCE
Alimentary tract and metabolism	Drugs for acid-related disorders	Dexlansoprazole, esomeprazole, famotidine, lansoprazole, omeprazole, pantoprazole
	Antiemetics and antinauseants	Meclizine, ondansetron
	Antidiarrheals, intestinal anti-inflammatory/anti-infective agents	Dicyclomine
	Drugs used for diabetes	Liraglutide, canagliflozin
	Vitamins	Calcium/cholecalciferol
Cardiovascular system	Cardiac therapy	Amiodarone
	Antihypertensives	Clonidine, doxazosin, guanfacine
	Diuretics	Hydrochlorothiazide/lisinopril, hydrochlorothiazide/losartan, hydrochlorothiazide/triamterene, hydrochlorothiazide/valsartan
	Peripheral vasodilators	Isosorbide, nitroglycerin
	Beta blockers	Atenolol, carvedilol, metoprolol
	Calcium channel blockers	Amlodipine, amlodipine/benazepril, diltiazem, verapamil
	Agents acting on the renin-angiotensin system	Benazepril, enalapril, lisinopril, losartan, ramipril, valsartan
	Lipid modifying agents	Fenofibrate, lovastatin
General anti-infectives	Antibacterials for systemic use	Ciprofloxacin, doxycycline, metronidazole
	Antimycotics for systemic use	Fluconazole
Genitourinary system and sex hormones	Sex hormones and modulators of the genital system	Progesterone, testosterone
	Urologicals	Oxybutynin, solifenacin, tamsulosin, terazosin
Musculoskeletal system	Anti-inflammatory and antirheumatic products	Celecoxib, diclofenac, meloxicam, ibuprofen, naproxen
	Muscle relaxants	Baclofen, cyclobenzaprine, carisoprodol, tizanidine

(continued)

Table 8-2 (continued). Drug Classes Associated With Commonly Dispensed Drugs Listing Xerostomia as a Potential Adverse Drug Reaction

ATC LEVEL 1 ANATOMIC GROUP	ATC LEVEL 2 THERAPEUTIC SUBGROUP	ATC LEVEL 5 CHEMICAL SUBSTANCE
Nervous system	Analgesics	Hydrocodone, morphine, oxycodone, sumatriptan, tramadol, acetaminophen/hydrocodone
	Antiepileptics	Carbamazepine, clonazepam, gabapentin, lamotrigine, pregabalin, topiramate
	Anti-Parkinson's drugs	Carbidopa/levodopa, ropinirole
	Psycholeptics	Alprazolam, aripiprazole, diazepam, hydroxyzine, quetiapine, risperidone, zolpidem
	Psychoanaleptics	Amitriptyline, bupropion, citalopram, donepezil, duloxetine, escitalopram, fluoxetine, lisdexamfetamine, methylphenidate, mirtazapine, nortriptyline, paroxetine, sertraline, trazodone, venlafaxine
	Other nervous system drugs	Dextroamphetamine/amphetamine
Respiratory system	Nasal preparations	Albuterol, albuterol/ipratropium, beclomethasone, fluticasone, fluticasone/salmeterol, mupirocin, triamcinolone
	Antiasthmatics	Budesonide/formoterol, ipratropium, mometasone, tiotropium
	Antihistamines for systemic use	Cetirizine, levocetirizine, loratadine, promethazine
Sensory organs	Ophthalmologicals	Brimonidine, dorzolamide/timolol

Adapted from ClinCalc (2018), Clinical Pharmacology (2018), and Lexicomp Online (2018).

The relationship between medications and xerostomia is tightly interwoven. First, the most common adverse effect associated with taking multiple medications (polypharmacy) is dry mouth (Dagli & Sharma, 2014). Second, the most frequently reported cause of dry mouth is xerostomic medications (Guggenheimer & Moore, 2003). With over 90% of adults taking at least one prescription medication and 40% of patients over 65 years old taking five or more prescriptions daily (Centers for Disease Control and Prevention, 2018), it is important for pharmacists to be aware of the occurrence and consequence of dry mouth and to provide alternatives for patients and prescribers.

According to Dagli and Sharma (2014), 1 in 9 U.S. citizens is over 60 years old, and this is projected to increase to 1 in 5 by the year 2050. With advancing age, older adults experience a greater number of comorbidities, which in turn results in an increase in the number of daily medications (Klotz, 2009). With the increase in medications, there is an analogous, or even exponential, increase in potential drug-related adverse reactions. Associated physiologic changes in aging, such as decreased lean body mass and serum albumin, can result in higher levels of unbound drugs in older adults (Lavan & Gallagher, 2016). Age-related pharmacokinetic changes in drug clearance can also result in potential toxicity-related drug reactions with decreased renal and hepatic clearance. The increased use of medications and comorbidities, along with a potentially increased risk of adverse events related to physiologic changes, results in older adults being at risk for developing xerostomia. Although aging does not have a negative impact on salivation (Ghezzi & Wagner-Lange, 2000), aging does result in salivary glands becoming more susceptible to the deleterious effects of disease and medication, and, thus, it is not surprising that xerostomia is the most frequently reported oral side effect among older adults.

It is estimated that 30% of the general population suffers from dry mouth. For patients with Sjögren's syndrome and for those undergoing radiation treatment for head and neck cancer, the incidence increases to 100% (Ship, 2003; Turner & Ship, 2007). If left untreated, xerostomia can lead to dental caries, dysgeusia, dysphagia, oral candidiasis, bacterial infection, halitosis, difficulty sleeping, oral lesions, and mastication problems (Ship, 2002; Tan, Lexomboon, Sandborgh-Englund, Haasum, & Johnell, 2018). Despite the high rate of incidence and potential complications, patients are frequently unaware that dry mouth is one of the most frequent adverse events associated with prescription and OTC medications. Therefore, pharmacists are in a unique position to help patients and providers identify potential drug-related causes of xerostomia and potential treatments. Table 8-3 includes a list of the drugs most frequently associated with xerostomia (but not necessarily the most commonly prescribed drugs). Drugs included in this list cause significant dry mouth in over 10% of patients (Wynn & Meiller, 2001) or have demonstrated higher levels of evidence of xerostomia as an adverse event in randomized clinical trials (Wolff et al., 2017). Table 8-3 is useful for pharmacists who have a medication history and want to determine the most likely causative agent of xerostomia.

In a report on managing xerostomia and salivary gland hypofunction, the American Dental Association Council on Scientific Affairs concluded that although the vast majority of medications do not damage salivary glands, there is a proportional increase in the likelihood of decreased unstimulated salivary flow rates as the number of comorbidities and the number of medications prescribed increase (Plemons, Al-Hashimi, & Marek, 2014). The use of multiple medications can lead to an increased number of ADRs either from the direct effect of the medication or from the interaction between medications (Sergi, De Rui, Sarti, & Manzato, 2011). Individuals taking more than four drugs are over 2.5 times more likely to experience an ADR than individuals taking fewer medications. The risk is even higher if the regimen includes diuretics, angiotensin-converting enzyme (ACE) inhibitors, or drugs for hypertension, which are some of the more common drug classes associated with xerostomia (Sergi et al., 2011). In a review of inappropriate prescribing patterns, Lavan and Gallagher (2016) found reports indicating patients taking two, four, or seven or more medications had a 13%, 38%, and 82% risk, respectively, of experiencing an ADR.

Xerostomia, in particular, is known to increase as the number of medications increases, making older adults especially vulnerable. Based on U.S. census data, there are 49.2 million citizens over age 65, which represents 15.2% of the U.S. population. This number is projected to increase to nearly 87 million citizens, representing 20% of the U.S. population, by the year 2050 (U.S. Census Bureau, 2018). According to the National Center for Statistics, the average person over 65 years old takes four to five medications, representing nearly two-thirds of all prescriptions dispensed (Kantor, Rehm, Haas, Chan, & Giovannucci, 2015). Older patients are more likely to be living with one or more chronic conditions that required multiple prescription and nonprescription treatments.

Table 8-3. Drugs Commonly Associated with Xerostomia

THERAPEUTIC SUBGROUP	DRUG NAME	> 10% INCIDENCE	HIGHER LEVEL EVIDENCE
Adrenergic agonist, bronchodilator	Isoproterenol	X	
Alpha-adrenergic receptor blocker	Guanabenz	X	
	Guanfacine	X	
	Reserpine	X	
Antiglaucoma	Brimonidine		X
Anti-anxiety agent, benzodiazepine	Alprazolam	X	
	Chlordiazepoxide	X	
	Clorazepate	X	
	Diazepam	X	
	Lorazepam	X	
	Oxazepam	X	
Antiarrhythmic	Propafenone	X	
Antiasthmatic	Tiotropium		X
Anti–bone-resorptive activity	Alendronate		X
Anticholinergic	Atropine	X	X
	Belladonna and opium	X	
	Benztropine	X	
	Diphenoxylate atropine	X	
	Glycopyrrolate	X	
	Hyoscyamine	X	
	Ipratropium	X	
	Methscopolamine	X	
Anticonvulsant	Clonazepam	X	
	Gabapentin		X
	Dimebon		X *(continued)*

Table 8-3 (continued). Drugs Commonly Associated with Xerostomia

THERAPEUTIC SUBGROUP	DRUG NAME	> 10% INCIDENCE	HIGHER LEVEL EVIDENCE
Antidepressant	Citalopram		X
	Duloxetine		X
	Escitalopram		X
	Fluoxetine		X
	Imipramine		X
	Nortriptyline		X
	Paroxetine		X
	Reboxetine		X
	Sertraline		X
	Sibutramine		X
	Venlafaxine	X	X
	Vortioxetine		X
Antidepressant, miscellaneous	Bupropion	X	X
	Nefazodone	X	
Antidepressant, MAOI	Phenelzine	X	
Antidepressant, SSRI	Paroxetine	X	X
Antidepressant, tricyclic	Amitriptyline	X	X
	Amoxapine	X	
	Clomipramine	X	
	Desipramine	X	
	Doxepin	X	
	Maprotiline	X	
	Protriptyline	X	
	Trimipramine	X	
Antiemetic	Nabilone	X	
	Prochlorperazine	X	
	Thiethylperazine	X	(continued)

Table 8-3 (continued). Drugs Commonly Associated with Xerostomia

THERAPEUTIC SUBGROUP	DRUG NAME	> 10% INCIDENCE	HIGHER LEVEL EVIDENCE
Antiglaucoma	Timolol		X
Antihistamine	Loratadine	X	
Antihypertensive/antiangina	Verapamil		X
Antihypertensive/antimigraine	Clonidine	X	X
Antinauseant/sedative/GI disorders	Scopolamine		X
Antineoplastic	Bevacizumab		X
Anti-Parkinson's	Rotigotine		X
	Selegiline	X	
Antiperistaltic/spasmolytic	Propantheline		X
Antipsychotic	Chlorpromazine		X
	Lithium		X
	Loxapine	X	X
	Molindone	X	
Antipsychotic	Perphenazine		X
	Risperidone		X
Antispasmodic	Dicyclomine	X	
Appetite suppressant	Phentermine		X
	Tesofensine		X
Atypical antipsychotic	Aripiprazole		X
	Clozapine		X
	Olanzapine		X
	Paliperidone		X
	Quetiapine		X *(continued)*

Table 8-3 (continued). Drugs Commonly Associated with Xerostomia

THERAPEUTIC SUBGROUP	DRUG NAME	> 10% INCIDENCE	HIGHER LEVEL EVIDENCE
Biological response modifier	Interferon alfa-2A	X	
	Interferon alfa-2B	X	
	Interferon alfa-N3	X	
Ergotamine	Ergot alkaloid	X	
Hypnotic agent	Doxylamine		X
Hypnotic agent, benzodiazepine	Estazolam	X	
	Quazepam	X	
	Temazepam	X	
Opioid analgesic	Butorphanol		X
	Buprenorphine		X
Psychostimulant–ADHD	Dexmethylphenidate		X
	Lisdexamfetamine		X
	Methylphenidate		X
Retinoic acid derivative	Isotretinoin	X	
Skeletal muscle relaxant	Baclofen		X
	Cyclobenzaprine	X	X
Strong diuretic	Furosemide		X
Urological–reduces bladder activity	Flavoxate	X	
	Imidafenacin		X
	Oxybutynin	X	X
	Propiverine		X
	Solifenacin		X
Urological–reduces bladder activity	Tolterodine		X
Weak diuretic	Bendroflumethiazide		X

Note: Wynn and Meiller (2001) identified drugs that cause significant dry mouth in more than 10% of patients. Wolff et al. (2017) reviewed published studies to identify drugs with a higher level of evidence.

ADHD = attention-deficit/hyperactivity disorder; GI = gastrointestinal; MAOI = monoamine oxidase inhibitor; SSRI = selective serotonin reuptake inhibitor.

In a study of community-dwelling older adults 65 to 95 years old, Smidt, Torpet, Nauntofte, Heegaard, and Pedersen (2011) observed a high prevalence for oral dryness was associated with metabolic, respiratory, and neurologic diseases and prescriptions for thyroid hormones, glucocorticoids, and other respiratory drugs. Antipsychotics (psycholeptics and/or psychoanaleptics), antineoplastics, proton pump inhibitors (PPIs), antidiabetic agents, loop diuretics, antispasmodics, quinine, and bisphosphonates were also associated with a high occurrence of dry mouth. Dry mouth is a common complaint in patients treated for hypertensive, psychiatric, or urinary problems and

Table 8-4. Comorbidities Commonly Seen in Patients Presenting With Xerostomia

- Dementia
- Diabetes
- Gastroesophageal reflux disease
- Head and neck cancer
- HIV/AIDS
- Hypertension
- Mental illness (e.g., depression, anxiety, psychosis)
- Neurodegenerative disorders (e.g., Parkinson's disease, fibromyalgia)
- Osteoporosis
- Pain and inflammation (e.g., muscular skeletal, rheumatoid arthritis, acute and chronic pain)
- Respiratory disorders (e.g., asthma, allergies)
- Sjögren's syndrome and other autoimmune diseases
- Urological disorders (e.g., urinary incontinence)

Adapted from Alsakran Altamimi (2014), Donaldson et al. (2014), Porter et al. (2004), Scully and Bagan (2004), Smidt et al. (2011), Tan et al. (2018), and Villa et al. (2015).

in older adults mainly because of the large number of drugs used and polypharmacy (Scully, 2003). The link between polypharmacy and dry mouth is both significant and strong.

Drugs within a therapeutic area (drug class) often share xerostomia as an adverse effect due to a common mechanism of action (Femiano et al., 2008). Table 8-2 presents a list of the therapeutic areas associated with the most commonly prescribed drugs that are associated with xerostomia, including urological drugs for urinary frequency and incontinence, antidepressants, antihypertensives, antihistamines, and psycholeptics. In addition, many of the drug classes known to cause xerostomia are the same ones associated with comorbidities common in older adults and/or associated with aging, such as hypertension, diabetes, Alzheimer's disease, muscle and joint pain, and Parkinson's disease (Villa, Connell, & Abati, 2015). In a review of randomized clinical trials associated with xerostomia in older adults, Tan et al. (2018) found the most commonly associated comorbidities included urinary incontinence; hypertension; cognitive impairment; insomnia; neuralgia; and mental health disorders, including major depression, generalized anxiety disorder, and psychosis. In a review of published studies pertaining to drug-related xerostomia from 2004 to 2014, Alsakran Altamimi (2014) identified associated comorbidities, including obesity, epilepsy, hypertension (diuretics), diarrhea, urinary incontinence, asthma (certain bronchodilators), and Parkinson's disease. The comorbidities most commonly treated with drugs that cause xerostomia and comorbidities that lead to xerostomia are included in Table 8-4 (Alsakran Altamimi, 2014; Donaldson, Epstein, & Villines, 2014; Porter et al., 2004; Scully & Bagan, 2004; Smidt et al., 2011; Tan et al., 2018; Villa et al., 2015).

PHARMACOLOGY

A review of the physiology associated with salivation is an important foundation to understand the pharmacology associated with medications that cause xerostomia and those that are used to treat symptoms associated with xerostomia. See Chapter 3 for a more detailed description of the parasympathetic and sympathetic divisions of the autonomic nervous system that are critical to the production of saliva. The role of acetylcholine and norepinephrine neurotransmitters and cholinergic, muscarinic, and adrenergic receptors in stimulating or suppressing salivation are also reviewed in Chapter 3.

Saliva is produced by the parotid, submandibular, and sublingual glands, as well as hundreds of minor submucosal salivary glands located throughout the mouth. Daily salivary output is estimated to be approximately 1 L/day, and flow rates can fluctuate by as much as 50% with circadian rhythm (Guggenheimer & Moore, 2003; Proctor, 2016).

A review of the mechanisms of action behind some of the drug classes known to be associated with xerostomia follows. Drug classes are grouped as having parasympathetic, sympathetic, or other mechanisms leading to a potential xerostomia ADR. Specific drugs within a drug class associated with xerostomia are provided. See the appendix at the end of this chapter for a comprehensive summary of all drugs (N > 500) listing xerostomia as a potential ADR (Clinical Pharmacology, 2018). Although the primary mechanism of drug-induced xerostomia is associated with anticholinergic activity or sympathomimetic action, some additional mechanisms associated with either xerostomia and/or reduced salivation flow include topical effects of inhaled medications, dehydration, vasoconstriction in salivary glands, alterations in electrolyte and fluid balance, changes in saliva composition, or direct damage to salivary glands (Sreebny & Schwartz, 1997; Tan et al., 2018).

Parasympathetic Pathways

The parasympathetic nervous system is essential for stimulating salivary gland secretion. As a result, drugs that interfere with the parasympathetic pathway will impact salivation. Salivary function can be inhibited by anticholinergic drugs at either the ganglionic (nicotinic) or acetylcholine receptors. Example ganglionic blocking agents are mecamylamine, trimethaphan, nicotine, and botulinum toxin type A and B. Salivary function can be inhibited by anticholinergic drugs at the muscarinic (acetylcholine) receptors on salivary acinar cells. Antihistamines (H1 receptor blockers), such as diphenhydramine, and tricyclic antidepressants (TCAs) are examples of drugs that show antimuscarinic activity (Sreebny & Schwartz, 1997).

Any drug that disrupts neurotransmission to salivary gland receptors or that interrupts ion transport pathways in salivary acinar cells can lead to salivary dysfunction. Drugs with anticholinergic or antimuscarinic activity are commonly associated with xerostomia and include anticholinergics, antipsychotics, antihistamines, and antimuscarinic drugs for urinary incontinence.

Anticholinergics

- Indication: Some indications include use as an antisialogogue preoperatively and interoperatively and as an antispasmodic postoperatively for nausea and vomiting and motion sickness.
- Mechanism: Atropine and scopolamine are high-affinity muscarinic antagonists known to reduce the secretions of many organs, including the salivary glands. Atropine functions as a sympathetic, competitive antagonist of muscarinic cholinergic receptors, thereby abolishing the effects of parasympathetic stimulation.
- Causative agents: Atropine, hyoscine (scopolamine)

Antihistamines

- Indication: Antihistamines reduce or block the effect of histamines and are used to alleviate symptoms associated with allergies.
- Mechanism: First-generation sedating H1 antihistamines are potent muscarinic receptor antagonists that can lead to serious anticholinergic side effects, such as dry mouth. Second-generation nonsedating antihistamines are more selective on peripheral H1 receptors and have a lower affinity for cholinergic and alpha-adrenergic receptor sites, which reduces the risk of anticholinergic and central nervous system side effects.
- Causative agents: Hydroxyzine, desloratadine, levocetirizine, fexofenadine, diphenhydramine, loratadine, cetirizine

Antipsychotics

- Indication: Phenothiazines, lithium, and other antipsychotic medications are used to treat schizophrenia, mood disorders, and other serious mental and emotional disorders. Dry mouth is one of the most common side effects with these medicines.
- Mechanism: Older, typical antipsychotics have a strong inhibiting effect on dopaminergic receptors and an affinity for muscarinic, histamine H1, or alpha-1 receptors, and are associated with frequent complaints of dry mouth. Newer, atypical antipsychotics have less robust, selective dopamine and serotonin 5HT-2 receptor blockade and less affinity for muscarinic, histaminergic, and alpha-adrenergic receptors. Atypical antipsychotics are less frequently associated with dry mouth and may be an alternative option for some patients. Dry mouth associated with lithium is reported to be as high as 70% in long-term treatment and is thought to result from a diuretic effect via inhibition of the action of the antidiuretic hormone in the kidney (Roganović, 2018).
- Causative agents:
  - Typical antipsychotics: Haloperidol, fluphenazine, decanoate, perphenazine, trifluoperazine, thiothixene, chlorpromazine, thioridazine, loxapine, molindone
  - Atypical antipsychotics: Clozapine, olanzapine, quetiapine, risperidone, tiapride
  - Other: Donepezil, lithium

Tricyclic Antidepressants

- Indication: TCAs are used to treat several types of depression and obsessive-compulsive disorder.
- Mechanism: TCAs enhance the actions of noradrenaline and serotonin by blocking their reuptake at the neuronal membrane, but they also block histaminic, alpha-1 adrenergic, and muscarinic cholinergic receptors, resulting in ADRs, such as dry mouth (Scully, 2003). As many as 70% to 85% of patients taking conventional TCAs report experiencing xerostomia (Roganović, 2018).
- Causative agents: Amitriptyline, clomipramine, desipramine, doxepin, imipramine, nortriptyline, protriptyline

Urinary Incontinence/Antimuscarinics

- Indication: Treat overactive bladder
- Mechanism: Most of the drugs used for urinary incontinence block muscarinic acetylcholine receptors, which can lead to dry mouth. The incidence for dry mouth in patients taking nonselective antimuscarinics is approximately 30% (Lam & Hilas, 2007). Patients suffering from dry mouth may find the extended-release formulations to cause less xerostomia. The M3-selective receptor antagonists may be more bladder specific and less prone to causing anticholinergic side effects, such as dry mouth. Mirabegron is a beta-3 adrenergic receptor agonist and may be an alternative for patients who are sensitive to dry mouth from antimuscarinic drugs (Tan et al., 2018).
- Causative agents
  - Nonselective antimuscarinics: Oxybutynin, tolterodine, and fesoterodine
  - M3-selective receptor antagonists: Darifenacin and solifenacin

Sympathetic Pathways

Patients who experience dry mouth as a result of drugs that alter the sympathetic nervous system may complain of a sticky feeling in their mouth, and their saliva may appear thick and ropy. Sympathetic blocking agents, such as chlorpromazine, ergotamine, and phentolamine, inhibit salivary flow by binding salivary alpha-1 adrenergic receptors (Sreebny & Schwartz, 1997). Drugs with sympathomimetic activity, such as ephedrine, alpha-1 antagonists (e.g., terazosin, prazosin), and alpha-2 agonists, may also reduce salivary flow. Beta blockers, especially nonselective agents with alpha-blocking effects, can change salivary protein levels and may result in xerostomia (Scully & Bagan, 2004). Other sympathomimetics that may serve as causative agents include decongestants, appetite suppressants, and bronchodilators.

Alpha-1 Blockers

- Indication: Bladder outlet obstruction associated with benign prostatic hyperplasia
- Mechanism: Blocking alpha-1 adrenergic receptors may alter saliva composition and secretion rates (Femiano et al., 2008). Alpha-1 agonists cause relaxation of the smooth muscle in the prostate and urethra. Postsynaptic alpha-1A adrenoceptors are also present in the salivary glands. Blockade of alpha-1 adrenoceptors in the salivary glands causes diminished excretion of water and potassium, which can lead to dry mouth (Netherlands Pharmacovigilance Centre Lareb, 2013). Tamsulosin binds selectively and competitively postsynaptic alpha-1A adrenoceptors and may be associated with less xerostomia compared with other less selective alpha blockers, such as terazosin (Scully, 2003).
- Causative agents: Tamsulosin, terazosin, doxazosin

Antidepressants

- Indication: Antidepressants are used to treat multiple types of depression and anxiety disorders as well as other conditions.
- Mechanism: Although SSRIs and selective serotonin–noradrenaline reuptake inhibitors can cause dry mouth, they are generally less likely to cause anticholinergic side effects than TCAs. The SSRIs selectively inhibit the reuptake of serotonin, and because they have little affinity for muscarinic or histamine receptors, they are associated with less pronounced xerostomia (Roganović, 2018; Tan et al., 2018). Bupropion is a selective reuptake inhibitor of dopamine and noradrenaline, and associated dry mouth is positively associated with metabolite concentration and inversely related to patient weight (Scully, 2003). Note that patients with anxiety or depressive conditions may report dry mouth even in the absence of drug therapy (Femiano et al., 2008; Scully & Felix, 2005).
- Causative agents:
  ◦ SSRIs: Escitalopram, paroxetine, fluoxetine, fluvoxamine, sertraline
  ◦ Norepinephrine reuptake inhibitor/selective serotonin–noradrenaline reuptake inhibitors: Duloxetine, venlafaxine, desvenlafaxine, reboxetine
  ◦ Aminoketone: Bupropion

Anti-HIV Drugs

- Indications: Didanosine is most commonly used along with other medications to treat HIV infection by decreasing the amount of HIV in the blood. Protease inhibitors are antiretroviral medicines that are most commonly used to prevent the HIV and hepatitis C viruses from multiplying in the body.
- Mechanism: The nucleoside reverse transcriptase inhibitor saquinavir mesylate is an inhibitor of the HIV protease. The exact mechanisms associated with xerostomia are unclear.
- Causative agents: Didanosine, saquinavir

Antihypertensives

- Indication: Antihypertensives are used to lower blood pressure but can be used for migraines and other conditions as well.
- Mechanism: Approximately 20% of patients with hypertension taking beta-adrenergic blockers report dry mouth. Beta blockers may decrease the total protein content of whole-mouth saliva (Femiano et al., 2008). The administration of ACE inhibitors may cause dry mouth due to the reduction of the salivary flow rate, whereas class 1 antiarrhythmic sodium channel blocker drugs are associated with dry mouth because of their anticholinergic effect (Femiano et al., 2008).
- Causative agents: Terazosin, prazosin, clonidine, atenolol, propranolol

Appetite Suppressants

- Indication: Appetite suppressants and weight loss
- Mechanism: The main side effects of sibutramine and other appetite suppressants, including dry mouth, are associated with its inherent sympathomimetic properties (Araújo & Martel, 2012).
- Causative agents: Sibutramine, fenfluramine plus phentermine, ephedrine

Benzodiazepines

- Indication: Benzodiazepines are used to treat anxiety disorders as well as other sedative and muscle relaxant conditions.
- Mechanism: Clinical trials link benzodiazepines to mild to moderate dry mouth. Animal studies have shown benzodiazepines decrease signaling molecules involved in muscarinic and alpha-1 adrenergic mediated salivary secretion (Roganović, 2018).
- Causative agents: Alprazolam, clonazepam, diazepam, lorazepam, clorazepate

Other Pathways

In addition to the sympathetic and parasympathetic autonomic nervous system, drugs may produce symptoms of xerostomia through other mechanisms. Examples include clonidine leading to salivary gland hypofunction by stimulating alpha-2 adrenoceptors in the frontal cortex, which in turn sends inhibitory signals to the salivary glands; diuretics contributing to a systemic loss of water, resulting in dehydration without any alteration in salivary flow rates; drugs leading to vasoconstriction of salivary gland vessels or causing changes in the composition of saliva secretions; and drug delivery systems, such as inhaled antiasthmatics, leading to xerostomia (Sreebny & Schwartz, 1997).

Antireflux Drugs

- Indication: H2 receptor antagonists and PPIs are used to reduce gastric acid secretion and promote healing associated with duodenal ulcers and gastroesophageal reflux disease.
- Mechanism: H2 receptor antagonists inhibit acid secretion by blocking H2 receptors on the parietal cell, and up to 41% of patients experience dry mouth (Scully & Bagan, 2004). PPIs suppress gastric acid secretion by inhibiting the hydrogen/potassium/ATPase enzyme system on the surface of the parietal cell.
- Causative agents:
  - PPIs: Omeprazole, esomeprazole, lansoprazole, pantoprazole, rabeprazole
  - H2 receptor antagonists: Famotidine, nizatidine

Cannabinoids

- Indication: Cannabinoids are most commonly used to treat neuropathic pain and spasticity, advanced cancer pain and nausea/vomiting, and as an appetite stimulant for patients with AIDS.
- Mechanism: Cannabis produces short-term hyposalivation due to tetrahydrocannabinol (Miranda-Rius, Brunet-Llobet, Lahor-Soler, & Farré, 2015). Cannabinoids bind to cannabinoid receptors in the submandibular saliva cells, inhibiting endocannabinoid stimulated salivation and modifying saliva content (Kopach et al., 2012).
- Causative agents: Medical marijuana

Cytotoxic Drugs and Cytokines

- Indication: Chemotherapy
- Mechanism: Direct damage to salivary glands
- Causative agents: Radioactive iodine, 5-fluorouracil, interleukin 2 (Scully, 2003; Ship, 2003)

Diuretics

- Indication: Diuretics are most commonly used to treat edema and hypertension.
- Mechanism: Dry mouth associated with diuretics is most likely related to dehydration or fluid depletion. Note that dehydration related to diabetes, chronic renal failure, hyperparathyroidism, or fever can also cause xerostomia.
- Causative agents: Furosemide, HCTZ

Opioids and Drugs of Abuse

- Indication: Pain
- Mechanism: Although there is a clear association between the use of opioids and dry mouth, the exact mechanism is unclear. Tramadol, a codeine analog, exerts its principal xerogenic effect by activating inhibitory pathways in the central nervous system and has no anticholinergic effect on the salivary glands at dosages that may be clinically relevant (Götrick & Tobin, 2004).

  Sympathomimetic drugs, such as cocaine and methamphetamine, mimic the actions of the endogenous neurotransmitters that stimulate the sympathetic nervous system, resulting in dry mouth. Over 70% of methamphetamine abusers experience xerostomia along with drug-induced bruxing and clenching, which can lead to severe tooth erosion and periodontal inflammation commonly known as *meth mouth* (Rommel et al., 2016).
- Causative drugs:
  - Opioids: Codeine, fentanyl, hydrocodone, hydromorphone, meperidine, methadone, morphine, oxycodone
  - Psychostimulants: Methamphetamine, cocaine

Oral Retinoids

- Indication: Most commonly used to treat acne vulgaris.
- Mechanism: Isotretinoin reduces salivary gland functions, salivary flow, and buffer capacity (Erdemir et al., 2017).
- Causative agents: Acitretin, isotretinoin

ROLE OF THE PHARMACIST

Pharmacists are in a unique position to assist patients experiencing dry mouth. Pharmacists can assist other health care providers (HCPs) and patients in identifying medications that may be causing xerostomia and in so doing prevent patients from taking their medications. Pharmacists can review medication histories and consult with prescribers to recommend alternative medications that do not cause, or are less likely to cause, xerostomia. If substitution is not possible, pharmacists can work with primary care providers to consider alternative dosing regimens or formulations. Finally, when medication changes are not an option, pharmacists can consult with patients and HCPs in identifying various treatment options including palliative self-care, saliva stimulants, saliva substitutes, or prescription sialogogues for more severe cases of xerostomia. Pharmacists in community settings are both knowledgeable and accessible to consumers to assist with information and treatment options for xerostomia. For patients suffering from autoimmune or radiation-induced xerostomia, pharmacists are available to consult with other HCPs regarding prescription therapies aimed at protecting mucosa or treating symptoms.

Medication History

In accordance with The Joint Commission (2019) medication reconciliation patient safety goals, pharmacists act as both advocates and medication experts to provide information and educate patients and HCPs. Specific elements to consider when taking a medication history for a patient with complaints pertaining to xerostomia might include the following:

- Review and assess the severity of symptoms: Villa et al. (2015) reviewed multiple questionnaires to assess dry mouth. Questions centered around rating perceived dryness of the mouth and lips, rating the difficulty associated with eating (especially dry foods) and swallowing, assessing if symptoms interfere with sleeping or speaking, and assessing actions the patient has already initiated to combat symptoms, such as sucking on candies and drinking water. See Chapter 2 for further discussion regarding starting a conversation about xerostomia with patients.

- Review existing medications and identify drugs that may be associated with xerostomia: See the appendix at the end of this chapter for a complete list of drugs with xerostomia listed as an ADR. See Table 8-3 for a list of drugs most commonly associated with xerostomia and Table 8-4 for a list of comorbidities whose associated drugs for treatment are most commonly associated with xerostomia.

- Review any OTC medications patients may be taking: OTC medications associated with xerostomia include those used to treat allergic conditions, congestion, motion sickness, acid reflux, and diarrhea.

- Review recreational drugs, including medical marijuana, which may be a contributing factor to xerostomia.

- Review medication administration: Identify options to reduce dose, reduce frequency, or avoid nighttime doses when salivary flow is normally at its lowest. Identify opportunities to discontinue medications known to cause xerostomia that are not critical for an existing comorbidity, recognizing that polypharmacy is associated with increased risk for xerostomia. Identify alternative medications less associated with dry mouth for any drugs identified during the medication history that are known to cause xerostomia.

- Provide patient education: Older patients on multiple medications, especially anticholinergics, are especially vulnerable to xerostomia. It is important to warn patients of potential decreases in the production of saliva because patients often do not notice symptoms until 50% of their normal saliva production is lost, which may be after the patient has suffered clinical consequences, such as enamel demineralization, caries, gingival disease, or halitosis (Sreebny & Schwartz, 1997).

- Obtain medical history: Identify any symptoms that may be consistent with associated auto-immune disease, such as Sjögren's syndrome, past or current salivary gland disorders (e.g., history of radiation treatment or head/neck trauma), or other risk factors, such as HIV infection. Assist patients in obtaining appropriate referrals.
- Emphasize the need for prevention: Reinforce the message that consistent, daily oral hygiene is critical to prevent dental caries and other disease progression; remind patients of the importance of a developing a strong therapeutic relationship with both their primary care provider and their dentist.
- Establish treatment strategy: Working with the patient, identify the best plan going forward regarding treatment strategies for symptom relief if causative factors cannot be eliminated.

TREATMENT STRATEGIES

Treatment options for symptoms associated with xerostomia include nonpharmacological palliative self-care strategies; saliva stimulants, which are particularly helpful for patients with intact salivary gland tissue; saliva substitutes, which are especially useful for patients without residual salivary function; and prescription sialogogues for patients with chronic or severe xerostomia.

Nonpharmacological General Treatment Strategies

General treatment strategies for the management and symptomatic relief of xerostomia consistent with recommendations from the American Academy of Oral Medicine are provided (Napeñas, Brennan, & Fox, 2009; Sankar & Rhodus, 2015). Readers are encouraged to cross-reference the following suggestions with the preceding chapters in which many of the recommendations are expanded upon.

1. Establish diagnosis: An interdisciplinary team may be necessary to establish a diagnosis and to work together to eliminate factors (e.g., medications) contributing to xerostomia (Turner & Ship, 2007).
2. Encourage all HCPs to complete an oral examination and discuss oral dryness with their patients.
3. Establish routine dental visits: Xerostomia is associated with an increased risk for dental caries, periodontal disease, and candidiasis. More frequent dental visits, including professional cleanings and in-office fluoride applications, may be required as a means of prevention.
4. Perform routine oral hygiene: Rinsing after each meal, brushing a minimum of two times per day, and flossing daily are recommended. Prescription-strength fluoride may be recommended. Meticulous, daily oral hygiene is one of the most important steps in successfully preventing and managing the complications of oral dryness.
5. Monitor mouth for oral candidiasis: Salivary gland hypofunction may alter normal flora, increasing the risk of opportunistic infections from organisms such as *Candida albicans*. Patients with a dry mouth should be advised to watch for signs of candidiasis (i.e., creamy, white bumps on the tongue or cheeks) and, if observed, to seek medical attention for evaluation and treatment (Nadig et al., 2017).
6. Avoid sugary food and drinks: To reduce further risk of dental caries, patients with xerostomia should be advised to decrease fermentable carbohydrate intake (e.g., cookies, cakes, soft drinks, bread, crackers, sweet breakfast cereal, bananas, dried fruits). Acidic beverages and sports drinks that can damage enamel should also be avoided.
7. Eat foods that require active mastication: For patients who do not have difficulty chewing, long root vegetables such as carrots and celery, as well as fresh apples, are recommended to engage active mastication, which promotes salivation.

8. Avoid caffeine: Caffeine is a mild diuretic that promotes fluid loss and may exacerbate dry mouth. Avoid coffee, tea, and soft drinks high in caffeine.

9. Stop tobacco use: Long-term smoking reduces the secretion and quality of saliva and increases xerostomia-related dental caries, gingivitis, tooth mobility, calculus, and halitosis (Petrušić, Posavac, Sabol, & Mravak-Stipetić, 2015; Rad, Kakoie, Niliye Brojeni, & Pourdamghan, 2010).

10. Avoid alcohol: Alcohol acts as a diuretic that promotes fluid loss and increases the risk for oral cancers (Seitz & Becker, 2007).

11. Frequently sip fluids or suck on ice: One of the easiest and least expensive ways to help relieve symptoms of xerostomia is to take frequent sips of small amounts of fluids, especially water. Letting chips of ice dissolve in the mouth or sucking on frozen grapes or sugarless popsicles may also be helpful. Note, however, that too much water can reduce the oral mucus film lining the mouth and worsen symptoms (Sankar & Rhodus, 2015).

12. Use fluids while eating: In addition to drinking liquids while eating, it may be helpful to add broth, sauces, gravy, or salad dressing to foods to soften and lubricate. These high-fat liquids also serve as additional calories for patients experiencing malnutrition secondary to xerostomia associated with head and neck radiation.

13. Protect dry lips: The use of regularly applied lip balms may provide soothing relief. The use of vitamin E–containing balm may also be helpful.

14. Use a humidifier: The use of a humidifier, especially at night, is recommended to prevent desiccating oral mucosa.

15. Breathe through your nose: Mouth breathing can lead to a more acidic oral environment that can cause or aggravate dry mouth. Changing your habit to nose breathing is encouraged if possible. Referral to an otolaryngologist may be advisable.

16. Avoid xerostomic OTC drugs: Some OTC products, including antihistamines, decongestants, PPIs, nasal inhalers, antidiarrheals, and antiemetics, may cause or exacerbate dry mouth.

17. Use alcohol-free mouth rinse formulated for dry mouth: There are numerous marketed mouthwashes that either soothe the mouth or help with remineralizing teeth to prevent dental caries. Some contain xylitol, which serves as both a sweetener and saliva stimulant. For most patients with dry mouth, mouth rinses that are alcohol free are preferred because alcohol also has a drying effect. There is little conclusive evidence to support the use of mouthwashes. The use of normal saline as a rinse is inexpensive and mildly antiseptic, but some patients may object to the taste. Sodium bicarbonate–based mouthwashes have mucolytic properties and could be helpful as a neutralizing agent. Some patients will object to the taste and may find the sodium bicarbonate to be an irritant. The use of chlorhexidine in mouthwashes serves as an antibacterial and antifungal agent and has antiplaque properties. Some patients may exhibit an allergic reaction, and cases of anaphylaxis have been reported. Chlorhexidine inactivates nystatin (which is prescribed to treat fungal infections) and can stain the teeth and tongue and be unpalatable. Products should be formulated as a 50:50 water:chlorhexidine solution. "Magic mouthwash" refers to compounded, prescription mouth rinses formulated to relieve symptoms from cancer-related oral complications. The formulations most frequently contain some combination of a topical analgesic agent, steroid, antifungal or antibacterial agent, and perhaps a mucosal coating agent. This mouthwash is often discussed on social media sites where patients with xerostomia exchange information.

18. Use toothpaste with fluoride: Toothpastes formulated for patients with dry mouth contain lower, or no, levels of sodium lauryl sulfate (SLS) and have low foaming activity to reduce the possibility of irritation. Look for formulations that contain fluoride, which is a naturally occurring mineral recognized for its ability to strengthen enamel and prevent dental caries.

Products that also contain calcium phosphopeptide–amorphous calcium phosphate may have additional remineralization properties. See Chapter 5 for more information on the use of prescription fluoride products/treatments. Some formulations also contain xylitol, a saliva stimulant. There are no randomized controlled studies comparing efficacy among products. Pharmacists should advise patients based on ingredients and cost and encourage patients to select products based on personal preference for texture and taste.

A representative list of toothpastes containing fluoride without a prescription include the following:

- ACT Dry Mouth Toothpaste (contains xylitol and is SLS free)
- Biotene Dry Mouth Fluoride Toothpaste, Original or Fresh Mint (SLS free)
- Colgate Hydris Dry Mouth Toothpaste (contains SLS)
- Premier Enamelon Fluoride Toothpaste (SLS free, contains stannous fluoride plus amorphous calcium phosphate remineralizing technology)
- Oral7 Moisturising Toothpaste (SLS free)
- Salivea Extra Gentle Toothpaste, Soothing Mint (contains xylitol and is SLS free)
- Smart Mouth Premium Toothpaste (contains SLS)
- TheraBreath Fresh Breath Toothpaste, Mild Mint (contains xylitol and is SLS free)

Saliva Stimulants

To the extent that functional salivary tissue remains, the regular use of sugar-free gum and lozenges is encouraged to help with mechanical and gustatory stimulation of saliva. Mints, lozenges, and gums can stimulate saliva secretion and reduce friction of the oral mucosa (Millsop, Wang, & Fazel, 2017). Salivation is also responsive to taste, particularly sour and bitter, and the use of flavored, sugar-free gums and lozenges increases secretory output and remains a mainstay of palliative therapy of xerostomia (Fox, 2004). Several studies on topical dry mouth products have found that patients with residual salivary function preferred chewing gum over other interventions. In a publication from the American Dental Association (ADA) on managing xerostomia and salivary gland hypofunction, sugar-free chewing gum is reported to be more helpful than other saliva substitutes; however evidence is insufficient to prove chewing gum is superior to other interventions in alleviating dry mouth symptoms (Plemons et al., 2014). Chewing gum or sucking on lozenges may enhance salivary flow routes, but these actions are likely to be transient.

Patients should be encouraged to look for products containing xylitol, which is a natural sweetener product that differs chemically from other sweeteners, such as sorbitol, fructose, and glucose and is not used by bacteria as a food source. Although xylitol is a U.S. Food and Drug Administration (FDA)–approved noncarcinogenic, zero-calorie, high-intensity sweetener, it also works to prevent tooth decay by interfering with the growth of bacteria (Hayes, 2001). Xylitol is generally well tolerated, although some patients may experience gastrointestinal disturbances, such as diarrhea or cramps, if xylitol-containing products are consumed in large (> 100 g daily) amounts (Mäkinen, 2016). A stick of gum generally contains 1 g xylitol. Note that although xylitol is safe and has a negligible effect on glucose in humans, it is harmful in canines. Patients should be advised to keep products away from animals. Sorbitol is another sugar substitute often found in gum but is less well tolerated. Patients should be advised to limit their consumption of sorbitol-containing gums and candies; as little as 10 g/day sorbitol (perhaps 5 to 10 candies or more) can cause diarrhea.

When consulting with patients on product selection, pharmacists should keep in mind that patients with head and neck cancer or patients who wear full dentures may find gum chewing difficult (Porter, 2004). Mints, lozenges, and candies should be allowed to dissolve slowly in the mouth. Candies with sugar should be avoided due to an increased risk of dental caries. Also, citrus-flavored or citric acid–containing candies should be used with caution because products with low pH may contribute to dental erosion (Frydrych, 2016). Products formulated to be more basic, and thus presumably less erosive, are XyliMelts discs and Salese lozenges (Delgado & Olafsson, 2017).

In working with patients to select a saliva stimulant, there are many formulation options to consider. Patients may need to try several products to find the formulation (gum vs. lozenge vs chew) and flavor most effective and appealing to them. Patients unable to chew may prefer a lozenge over the use of gum or chewable products. Patients who have the greatest need for saliva stimulation during sleep may find XyliMelts discs, which are designed to adhere to the vestibule area of the mouth, to be a convenient option and are safe for nighttime use as well as during the day. The adherence of the disc provides a time-release function, resulting in longer-lasting relief compared with other saliva stimulants. Others may find adhesive properties, or some flavorings, to be irritating. Size is yet another factor because some lozenges are larger than others and may interfere with speaking. The cost of products may also be a factor, especially for patients seeking long-term therapy options.

A representative list of xylitol-containing saliva stimulant formulations and products follows:

- Lozenge/mint
  - ACT Dry Mouth Lozenges, Mint or Honey
  - Hager Pharma Dry Mouth Drops with Xylitol, Assorted Pack
  - Nutra BioGenesis Xylitol Peppermint Mints
  - OraCoat XyliMelts Discs for Dry Mouth, Mild Mint or Mint Free
  - Nature's Sweet Life Xylitol Mints
  - Ricochet Fruit Sours and Mints
  - Salese Sensitive, Hours of Dry Mouth Relief, Moisturizing Lozenges, Mild Lemon
  - SmartMouth Dry Mouth Dual-Action Mints
  - Solaray Mini Mints
  - Spry Mints
  - Thayers Sugar-Free Citrus Dry Mouth Lozenges
  - TheraBreath Sugar-Free Dry Mouth Lozenges, Mandarin Mint
  - TheraMints (3M)
  - Xylichew Mints
  - Xponent Xylitol Mints
- Gum
  - ACT Dry Mouth Gum
  - Biotene Dry Mouth Gum (also contains sorbitol)
  - Epic Xylitol Gum
  - Orbit Sugarfree Gum
  - Ricochet Gum
  - Spry Gum with 100% Xylitol
  - TheraBreath ZOX Mints
  - Trident Gum with Xylitol (also contains sorbitol)
  - Xponent Xylitol Gum
  - XyloBurst
  - Zapp! Gum
- Chews
  - BasicBites (chocolate flavor)

Saliva Substitutes

Healthy humans secrete between 0.5 and 2.0 L saliva per day. Natural saliva is slightly alkaline, with resting saliva having a pH between 5.7 and 6.2. Stimulated saliva can reach a pH as high as 8.0 (Kubala et al., 2018). Natural saliva contains organic and inorganic substances suspended in an aqueous medium. Saliva is 99% water but also contains glycoproteins (e.g., mucin), digestive enzymes (e.g., lipase, amylase), and various electrolytes (Kubala et al., 2018). Other compounds, such as lactoferrins, cystatin, histatin, thiocyanate ion, immunoglobulins, and lipids, are also present (Preetha & Banerjee, 2005).

Saliva has several distinct functions including cleansing, lubrication, maintaining mucosal integrity, buffering, remineralization, digestion, and antimicrobial activity. Along with muscle activity, saliva washes away the food particles from the oral mucosa by moving debris from teeth and soft tissues progressively toward the back of the mouth. Eventually, swallowing occurs. Glycoproteins in saliva are responsible for the viscoelastic character, giving it a lubricative film, which enables free movement of oral tissues and aids in speech (Preetha & Banerjee, 2005). Mucin and electrolytes contribute to the hydration of the oral mucosa, providing mucosal integrity.

The most prominent buffering agents in saliva are bicarbonate and phosphate ions; these agents protect the dentition from demineralization. Ions such as phosphate, calcium, and fluoride help for the remineralization of teeth by promoting surface binding to the hydroxyapatite surface, restoring those leached substances to tooth enamel. Enzymes like amylase and lipase initiate fat degradation and break down select starches into maltose and dextrin, thus serving a role in the digestion function. The antimicrobial, antiviral, and antifungal activity of saliva is due to the presence of lactoferrins, immunoglobulins, cystatin, histatin, thiocyanate ions, and lubricating mucins (Kubala et al., 2018). Although proteins and electrolytes only account for 1% of the contents of saliva, the loss of these organic and inorganic constituents that are essential to inhibiting cariogenic microorganisms and buffering oral acids can lead to an acceleration of tooth decay (Guggenheimer & Moore, 2003; Ship, 2003).

To combat adverse effects related to reduced salivation, several saliva substitutes have been formulated. Although artificial saliva is not an exact replacement for the saliva produced naturally by salivary glands, the combination of ingredients can help relieve symptoms. The ideal saliva substitute (a) would be long lasting, (b) provide lubrication to protect the oral mucosa, (c) promote bactericidal activity to prevent dental caries, and (d) be associated with a high level of patient acceptance regarding taste and mouth feel. Unfortunately, salivary substitutes are generally not well accepted by patients, and they are removed from the mouth during swallowing. As a result, they have a short duration of action and only provide relief for a short period of time.

Saliva substitutes function in improving lubrication and hydration of oral tissues and maintaining oral health and function (Porter et al., 2004). The present saliva substitutes do not serve as substitutes for the digestive and enzymatic actions of natural saliva; however, they are formulated to be as close as possible to natural saliva in terms of chemical composition and biophysical properties (Villa et al., 2015).

Common ingredients in artificial saliva are water and a combination of the following ingredients:

- Viscosity agents: Carboxymethylcellulose and hydroxyethyl cellulose are used as thickening agents to increase the viscosity of formulations and lubricate the oral cavity. Glycerin is a colorless, odorless lipid. In artificial saliva, glycerin coats the tongue, teeth, and gums to reduce moisture loss and protect the mouth from mechanical trauma. Natural mucins, such as porcine gastric mucin and bovine submandibular mucin, simulate the viscoelastic properties of human saliva (Nieuw Amerongen & Veerman, 2003).
- Minerals: Minerals, such as fluoride, calcium chloride, and phosphate ions, are added to inhibit demineralization and enhance remineralization. Some products also contain zinc or cetylpyridinium chloride to prevent gingivitis.
- Preservatives: Propyl paraben or methyl paraben are used to maintain shelf life.

- Flavoring: Flavoring agents, such as mint, sorbitol, or xylitol, are added for palatability. Xylitol is also used to stimulate saliva production and to protect teeth from bacteria and prevent dental caries.

In a comparison of saliva substitutes, patients rated gel formulations as performing the best; yet, they selected the carboxymethylcellulose spray as their favorite compound based on taste and ease of handling (Momm, Volegova-Neher, Schulte-Mönting, & Guttenberger, 2005). Patient preferences are highly variable, and although pharmacists can make recommendations based on the dosage form and formulation of ingredients, ultimately preference and use will be determined by factors such as taste, texture, compatibility of dosage form with patient lifestyle, and cost.

Despite several options for saliva stimulation and saliva substitution, a review of randomized clinical trials indicates there is no strong evidence that any one option is particularly effective or better than any other. Patient satisfaction with saliva substitutes is low. Although saliva substitutes can provide some symptomatic relief, none of the options are as effective as saliva (Frydrych, 2016; Furness, Worthington, Bryan, Birchenough, & McMillan, 2011). Although saliva substitutes do provide relief for patients suffering from radiation-induced xerostomia, they are generally not tolerated due to a short duration of action, undesirable taste (slimy mouth feel), inconvenience, and high cost (Radvansky, Pace, & Siddiqui, 2013).

When considering/comparing products, look for products containing xylitol, such as Mouth Kote or Oasis Moisturizing Mouth Spray, or ones containing carboxymethylcellulose or hydroxyethyl cellulose, such as Biotene Oral Balance. Saliva substitutes that contain fluoride and are supersaturated with calcium and phosphate are the most effective to prevent demineralization and to foster tooth remineralization (Hahnel, Behr, Handel, & Bürgers 2009). If the saliva substitute does not contain fluoride, consider concomitant use of a fluoride rinse.

See Table 8-5 for a partial list of saliva substitutes, including key ingredients. The products included are grouped by formulation type. The comparative list of ingredients, along with patient preferences and experiences regarding taste, formulation, and cost can be used in assisting patients with product selection.

Saliva substitutes are short acting and are most effective when applied before sleeping and speaking. The frequency of use varies based on the severity of patient symptoms. Generally, saliva substitutes are used three to five times per day or whenever dry mouth becomes uncomfortable. Patients suffering from xerostomia secondary to radiation may require application up to 10 times per day. Additional patient education messages for patients should include the following:

- Oral rinses are generally not meant to be swallowed (ingesting small amounts is not toxic). Patients should swish small amounts orally for 30 seconds and then spit out.
- High-concentration mineral powders should be diluted in about 1 oz water before swishing for 30 seconds and spitting out. Solution is not preserved and should not be stored once it is reconstituted.
- Oral sprays, as well as gels, pastes, or swabs, can be applied directly to the oral cavity. Patients should be advised to follow package instructions regarding storage. Package instructions will also contain directions regarding shaking of liquid sprays, if required.

Sialogogues and Other Systemic Treatments

Secretagogues are substances that stimulate secretions. Sialogogues are a specific type of secretagogue that stimulate the flow of saliva. The most common prescription sialogogues approved by the FDA for use in treating dry mouth, primarily due to Sjögren's syndrome or radiation therapy, are pilocarpine and cevimeline. Both of these agents are strong cholinergic, parasympathetic agonists and are generally well tolerated. In a report issued by the American Dental Association, the authors concluded the following:

Table 8-5. Comparative Ingredients for Representative Saliva Substitute Products

FORMULATION AND PRODUCT NAME	VISCOSITY BASE	XYLITOL	SORBITOL	FLUORIDE	CALCIUM	ENZYMES	CPC	ZINC	PHOSPHATES
Gel									
Biotene Oralbalance Moisturizing Gel	HEC/glycerin	X	X						
GC Dry Mouth Gel	CMC/polyglycerol								
Oral7 Moisturising Mouth Gel	HEC/glycerin	X	X			X			
BioXtra Dry Mouth Gel	HEC/glycerin	X	X			X			
Liquid									
ACT Dry Mouth Anticavity Fluoride Mouthwash	Glycerin	X	X	X	X				X
Biotene Dry Mouth Oral Rinse	HEC	X	X						X
Colgate Hydris Oral Rinse for Dry Mouth	Glycerin/XG		X				X		X
Crest Pro-Health Rinse	Glycerin						X		
Oasis Moisturizing Mouthwash	Glycerin/XG		X				X		X
Salivea Dry Mouth Care Extra Gentle Mouthwash	HEC/glycerin	X			X	X		X	X
SmartMouth Dry Mouth Activated Oral Rinse	CMC/glycerin							X	
TheraBreath Dry Mouth Oral Rinse	CMC/glycerin	X				X			

(continued)

Table 8-5 (continued). Comparative Ingredients for Representative Saliva Substitute Products

FORMULATION AND PRODUCT NAME	VISCOSITY BASE	XYLITOL	SORBITOL	FLUORIDE	CALCIUM	ENZYMES	CPC	ZINC	PHOSPHATES
Liquid									
MoiStir (Kingswood Labs)	CMC/ glycerin		X		X				X
Numoisyn	Linseed oil		X						X
Spray									
ACT Dry Mouth Spray	Glycerin/ PEG	X	X		X				X
Allday Dry Mouth Spray (Epic)	Glycerin/ glycol	X							
Biotene Dry Mouth Moisturizing Spray	Glycerin/ PEG/XG	X					X		
Lubricity Spray	Sodium hyaluronate	X							
Mouth Kote Remint Remineralizing Dry Mouth Spray (Parnell Pharmaceutical)	Yerba santa	X	X	X					

(continued)

Table 8-5 (continued). Comparative Ingredients for Representative Saliva Substitute Products

FORMULATION AND PRODUCT NAME	VISCOSITY BASE	XYLITOL	SORBITOL	FLUORIDE	CALCIUM	ENZYMES	CPC	ZINC	PHOSPHATES
Spray									
Oasis Mouth Moisturizing Spray for Dry mouth	Glycerin/PEG/XG	X					X		
Salivea Hydrating Mouth Spray Gentle Mint	XG/PEG	X				X			
Stoppers 4 Dry Mouth Spray	HEC/glycerin	X				X			
TheraBreath Fresh Breath Throat Spray	PEG	X	X					X	
Aquae Dry Mouth Spray (Amcal)	CMC	X			X				
AS Saliva Orthana Spray	Mucin	X							
BioXtra Dry Mouth Gel Mouthspray	HEC	X	X	X	X	X			X
Glandosane Artificial Saliva Spray	CMC		X		X				X
Prescription Super Saturated Calcium									
NeutraSal (powder for reconstitution)	n/a				X				X
SalivaMax (powder for reconstitution)	n/a				X				X
Caphosol solution (EUSA Pharma)	n/a				X				X
3M Xerostomia Relief Spray	OGT								
Aquoral solution	OGT								

CMC = carboxymethylcellulose; CPC = cetylpyridinium chloride; HEC = hydroxyethyl cellulose; OGT = oxidized glycerol triesters; PEG = polyethylene glycol; XG = xanthan gum.

Response to these medications may vary based on the amount of healthy acinar cells within the salivary glands. Patients with extensive salivary gland damage, such as those with radiation-induced SGH [salivary gland hypofunction], may not respond as well as do patients with less severe damage. (Plemons et al., 2014, pp 13-14)

Additional systemic medications indicated for use in xerostomia include amifostine (Ethyol), which is a cytoprotective agent used during radiation to treat associated radiation-induced xerostomia, and Sialor (anethole trithione), which is an OTC saliva stimulant available in Canada.

Other compounds that are reported to increase salivary flow but are not specifically approved for use in treating xerostomia include bethanechol, bromhexine, pyridostigmine, yohimbine, and interferon (Fox, 2004; Kavitha, Mubeen, & Vijayalakshmi, 2017). Complementary and alternative medicines are also reviewed briefly. Drug information sources include manufacturer label information approved by the FDA, Lexicomp (2018), and additional sources as cited.

Pilocarpine (Salagen Tablets)

- Pharmacology (mechanism of action): Pilocarpine is a potent cholinergic agonist that acts directly on muscarinic receptors to stimulate secretion by exocrine glands (i.e., salivary, sweat, lacrimal, gastric, pancreatic, intestinal, and respiratory mucous cells) and to increase smooth muscle tone (e.g., gastrointestinal tract, bronchi, urinary tract, gall bladder, and biliary tract).

  Systemic pilocarpine is approved for the management of xerostomia secondary to radiation-induced salivary gland damage and for dry mouth associated with Sjögren's syndrome. Pilocarpine may also be of benefit in treating drug-induced dry mouth, particularly if there is an associated decrease in salivary flow (Wilcock, Twycross, Mortimer, & Thresiamma, 2006).

  Numerous randomized clinical trials have demonstrated the effectiveness of systemic pilocarpine on dry mouth and salivary function in patients with Sjögren's syndrome and postradiation salivary gland hypofunction (Fox, 2004).

- Pharmacokinetics: Pilocarpine is readily absorbed from the gastrointestinal tract with a 20-minute onset of action, a peak plasma concentration in approximately 1 hour, and a 3- to 5-hour duration of action. A high-fat diet decreases the rate of absorption and time to peak concentration. Pilocarpine is metabolized by CYP2A6 in the liver and is excreted principally by means of the kidneys, with the elimination half-life being approximately 1 hour (Porter et al., 2004). Patients with a 30% decrease in liver function will experience higher peak plasma concentrations and a doubling of exposure due to a longer period of time for drug clearance. Dosage adjustment is recommended in patients with moderate hepatic impairment. Manufacturer labeling does not specify dosage adjustment in renal insufficiency. Pilocarpine is not protein bound. Increases in salivary secretion are dose dependent. Patients do not develop a tolerance to the secretagogue effects of pilocarpine (Fox, 2004).

- Interactions (drugs, dietary supplements, food, laboratory, and disease): There are no specific drug interactions requiring avoidance of concomitant use. The cholinergic effects of pilocarpine may be increased and should be considered before prescribing an acetylcholinesterase inhibitor. Caution should also be used when giving pilocarpine to patients taking beta-adrenergic antagonists (beta blockers) because of the possibility of cardiovascular conduction disturbances.

- Dose and routes of administration: The recommended initial dose of pilocarpine for patients suffering from xerostomia related to radiation-induced salivary gland damage is 5 mg three times/day. The dose can be titrated based on response and tolerability. The usual, effective dose is 15 to 30 mg/day (not to exceed 10 mg/dose and not to exceed 30 mg/day). Although improvement may be seen quickly, at least 12 weeks of continuous therapy is recommended to determine effectiveness. For patients suffering from xerostomia related to Sjögren's syndrome, the recommended dose is 5 mg four times/day with similar titration as needed.

  Although pilocarpine is well tolerated, common side effects are dose related, and patients should be dosed at the lowest effective dose for maintenance treatment. Dose adjustment is not specified for mild hepatic disease or rental insufficiency. A reduced starting dose of 5 mg two times/day and titration upward to 5 mg three to four times/day as tolerated is recommended for patients with moderate to severe hepatic involvement.

- Contraindications and precautions: Pilocarpine is contraindicated in patients with uncontrolled asthma, when miosis would exacerbate disease, such as acute iritis or narrow-angle glaucoma, and when there is known hypersensitivity to pilocarpine.

  Pilocarpine should be used with caution in patients with respiratory disorders, such as controlled asthma, chronic bronchitis, or chronic obstructive pulmonary disease due to the potential for increased airway resistance, bronchial smooth muscle tone, and bronchial secretions.

  Pilocarpine should be used with caution in patients with cardiovascular disease because they may be unable to compensate for transient changes in hemodynamics or rhythm induced by pilocarpine.

  Patients with cholelithiasis, biliary tract disease, and/or nephrolithiasis should use pilocarpine with caution due to the potential for smooth muscle spasms, which could precipitate complications such as cholecystitis, biliary obstruction, or renal colic or ureteral reflux.

  Pilocarpine has a category C pregnancy classification. Although the FDA has implemented a new pregnancy rating system, the older category C rating was defined as follows: animal reproduction studies have shown an adverse effect on the fetus and there are no adequate and well-controlled studies in humans, but potential benefits may warrant use of the drug in pregnant women despite potential risks.

- ADRs: Clinical experience to date suggests that pilocarpine is safe and well tolerated, and serious adverse events are rare (Porter et al., 2004). Although side effects such as sweating, flushing, and urinary frequency are common, they are typically of mild or moderate intensity and of relatively short duration (Wiseman & Faulds, 1995).

  As a nonselective muscarinic agonist, pilocarpine acts to increase secretions not only on salivary glands but also on all exocrine glands throughout the body. As a result, one of the main side effects of pilocarpine is an increased amount of sweating (Fox, 2004). Other common side effects occurring in greater than 10% of patients include flushing, chills, dizziness, headache, nausea, urinary frequency, rhinitis, and weakness. Less frequent side effects occurring between 1% and 10% include edema, hypertension, palpitation, tachycardia, pain, fever, somnolence, pruritus, rash, diarrhea, dyspepsia, vomiting, constipation, flatulence, glossitis, stomatitis, taste perversion, vaginitis, myalgia, tremor, ocular lacrimation, amblyopia, abnormal vision, blurred vision, conjunctivitis, tinnitus, cough, dysphagia, epistaxis, sinusitis, allergic reaction, and voice alteration.

- Monitoring parameters for efficacy and toxicity: Clinical trials have used symptoms of dry mouth as the primary outcome variable. Additional studies measuring the impact of pilocarpine on improving xerostomia and reducing dental caries would be valuable. Secondary variables included the amount of salivary output, other oral dryness symptoms, and patients' perceptions of oral functioning (Fox, 2004).

- Patient education messages: Patients should be informed that if a dose is missed, the next dose should be taken at the next regularly scheduled time (i.e., do not double up on a dose to make up for a missed dose). Tablets can be taken with or without food (except high-fat meals).

  If a patient sweats excessively while taking pilocarpine and they cannot drink enough liquid, they should consult a physician to avoid dehydration.

  Although less common with oral (vs. optic) pilocarpine, visual disturbances can occur, especially at night, and patients should be cautious until they know how pilocarpine affects their ability to drive.

- Cost of therapy: Pilocarpine 4% eye drops may be less expensive than tablets. Eye drops can be taken orally (three to five drops three times/day placed on tongue [6 to 10 mg pilocarpine]) if tablets are not covered by insurance or swallowing is an issue. The maximum dose is 10 mg/dose and 30 mg/day (Wilcock et al., 2006). Pilocarpine is available in an ophthalmic solution, a gel, and as an oral tablet (Salagen). The tablet can also be compounded into an oral solution of varying concentrations.

According to Goodrx.com (n.d.a.), at the time of this publication, a 90-day supply of pilocarpine tablets 5 mg four times/day retails from $50.15 to an average retail cost of $138.87.

Cevimeline (Evoxac Capsules)

- Pharmacology (mechanism of action): Cevimeline is a cholinergic agonist that selectively binds to M1 and M3 muscarinic receptors located on lachrymal and salivary gland epithelium. As opposed to pilocarpine, cevimeline has less affinity for M2 and M4 receptors located on cardiac and lung tissues and therefore can enhance salivary secretion while minimizing pulmonary and cardiac involvement (Ship, 2003). Cevimeline increases the secretion of salivary and sweat glands and the tone of the smooth muscle in the gastrointestinal and urinary tracts. Cevimeline is approved for use in treating dry mouth associated with Sjögren's syndrome and is well tolerated at recommended doses.

- Pharmacokinetics: Cevimeline is readily absorbed from the gastrointestinal tract with a mean time to peak concentration of 1.5 to 2 hours. When administered with food, there is a decreased rate of absorption and time to peak concentration. Cevimeline is metabolized by CYP2A6 and CYP3A3/4 in the liver and is excreted principally by means of the kidneys, with the elimination half-life being approximately 5 hours. Manufacturer labeling does not specify dosage adjustment in hepatic or renal insufficiency. Cevimeline is less than 20% protein bound.

- Interactions (drugs, dietary supplements, food, laboratory, disease): Analogous to pilocarpine, there are no specific drug interactions requiring avoidance of concomitant use. The cholinergic effects of cevimeline may be pronounced when taken in combination with other acetylcholinesterase inhibitors. Cevimeline should also be administered with caution to patients taking beta-adrenergic antagonists because of the possibility of conduction disturbances.

Drugs that inhibit CYP2D6 and CYP3A3/4 also inhibit the metabolism of cevimeline. Cevimeline should be used with caution in individuals known or suspected to be deficient in CYP2D6 activity, based on previous experience, because they may be at a higher risk of adverse events.

- Dose and routes of administration: The recommended dose of cevimeline hydrochloride is 30 mg taken three times a day. At the time of approval, there was insufficient safety information to support doses greater than 30 mg three times a day as well as insufficient evidence for additional efficacy at doses greater than 30 mg three times/day. Subsequent studies have demonstrated that cevimeline is efficacious at both 30 mg three times a day and 60 mg three times a day, but patients experience a great occurrence of gastrointestinal tract disorders at the higher dose (Fife et al., 2002; Porter et al., 2004).

- Contraindications and precautions: Similar to pilocarpine, cevimeline is contraindicated in patients with uncontrolled asthma, known hypersensitivity to cevimeline, acute iritis, and narrow-angle (angle-closure) glaucoma when miosis would lead to additional complications.

Cevimeline should be used with caution in patients with a history of cardiovascular disease because cevimeline may alter cardiac conduction and/or heart rate. Similar to pilocarpine, patients taking cevimeline may not be able to compensate for transient hemodynamic changes or changes in heart rate.

Cevimeline should be used with caution in patients with respiratory disorders such as controlled asthma, chronic bronchitis, or chronic obstructive pulmonary disease due to the potential for increased airway resistance, bronchial smooth muscle tone, and bronchial secretions.

Patients with cholelithiasis, biliary tract disease, and/or nephrolithiasis should use cevimeline with caution due to the potential for smooth muscle spasms, which could precipitate complications such as cholecystitis or biliary obstruction, renal colic, or ureteral reflux.

Cevimeline is classified as an FDA pregnancy category C drug.

- ADRs: Clinical experience to date suggests that cevimeline is safe and generally well tolerated with minimal adverse cardiac and pulmonary effects due to its selective affinity for muscarinic receptors on salivary and sweat glands (Ship, 2003).

  Based on clinical trials submitted for drug approval, the most common muscarinic-associated adverse events (> 10%) include excessive sweating, nausea, rhinitis, and diarrhea.

  Less common adverse reactions associated with cevimeline occurring between 1% and 10% include excessive salivation, urinary frequency, asthenia, flushing, and polyuria.

- Monitoring parameters for efficacy and toxicity: There are no specific laboratory tests or monitoring parameters required for patients treated with cevimeline. Cevimeline toxicity is characterized by an exaggeration of its parasympathomimetic effects including headache, visual disturbance, lacrimation, sweating, respiratory distress, gastrointestinal spasm, nausea, vomiting, diarrhea, atrioventricular block, tachycardia, bradycardia, hypotension, hypertension, shock, mental confusion, cardiac arrhythmia, and tremors.

- Patient education messages: Patients should be informed that if a dose is missed, the next dose should be taken at the next regularly scheduled time (do not double up on a dose to make up for a missed dose).

  Patients who sweat excessively should be advised to drink extra water and consult with a primary care provider because cevimeline can cause dehydration.

- Cost of therapy: According to Goodrx.com (n.d.b.), at the time of this publication, a 90-day supply of cevimeline capsules 30 mg three times/day retails from $87.17 to an average retail cost of $265.53.

Amifostine (Ethyol for Injection)

Amifostine powder for reconstitution is a radioprotective drug approved for use in reducing moderate to severe xerostomia due to radiation therapy associated with head and neck cancer. For maximum effectiveness, patients must have a substantial portion of parotid glands in the radiation field. Used in combination with radiotherapy, Gu et al. (2014) reported that amifostine significantly reduces the side effects of serious mucositis, acute/late xerostomia, and dysphagia. Other reviews find amifostine-related improvement to be less significant (Miranda-Rius et al., 2015). The most common amifostine-related side effects seen in clinical studies were nausea, emesis, hypotension, and allergic responses (Jensen et al., 2010). The reduction of radiation-induced toxicities by amifostine should be weighed against the toxicities of amifostine itself according to the individual treatment strategy (Gu et al., 2014).

Anethole Trithione (Sialor) Tablets

Anethole trithione is an OTC saliva stimulant available in Canada and on prescription in some other countries outside the United States. Anethole trithione is a bile secretion–stimulating drug or cholagogue. Anethole increases the availability of muscarinic receptors, resulting in the stimulation of salivary acinar cells (Porter et al., 2004). Anethole has been used in drug-induced and radiation-induced xerostomia as well as xerostomia in patients with Sjögren's syndrome but with conflicting reports on efficacy (Fox, 2004; Porter et al., 2004). Anethole comes as a 25-mg tablet, and the recommended dose is 25 mg three times/day before meals.

Bethanechol

Bethanechol is a muscarinic antagonist that has been shown to increase unstimulated and stimulated salivary flow rates in patients with xerostomia secondary to radiation (Porter et al., 2004). More recent studies have demonstrated positive symptomatic improvement after 3 weeks in patients treated with 25 mg bethanechol three times/day (Kavitha et al., 2017). Adverse events were not significant, which is consistent with other reviews of bethanechol for xerostomia (Kavitha et al., 2017; Porter et al., 2004).

Bromhexine

Bromhexine may increase salivary and lacrimal flow in patients with Sjögren's syndrome and result in some symptomatic relief of radiation-induced xerostomia, but studies are limited and generally find that other therapeutics agents, such as pilocarpine, are more effective (Abbasi, Farhadi, & Esmaili, 2013; Porter et al., 2004).

Pyridostigmine and Yohimbine

Pyridostigmine and yohimbine have been suggested as potential agents to provide benefit in the treatment of drug-related xerostomia, but randomized controlled trials to confirm efficacy are lacking (Porter et al., 2004).

Interferon Alpha

Injectable interferon alpha is a recombinant protein that has been tested in several large clinical trials as both a high-dose injectable and a low-dose lozenge for xerostomia in patients with Sjögren's syndrome. Interferon alpha was well tolerated and may have potential in improving salivary gland function (Fox, 2004).

Infliximab and Rituximab

Infliximab is a tumor necrosis factor inhibitor, and rituximab is a monoclonal antibody targeting B lymphocytes. Both agents are disease-modifying antirheumatic drugs that have been investigated for potential use in treating patients with Sjögren's syndrome. An increased salivary flow rate and patient-reported symptomatic improvement have been observed in some studies (Fox, 2004; Miranda-Rius et al., 2015).

Complementary and Alternative Medicines

Herb-based preparations and essential fatty acids, including jaborandi (which contains pilocarpine), betel nut (which contains arecoline, a muscarinic agonist), bakumondoto, Iceland moss (*Cetraria islandica*), evening primrose oil, alpha-linolenic acid, and Longo Vital have all been reported to stimulate salivary secretion, although significance has not been established (Fox, 2004; Miranda-Rius et al., 2015).

Medications are the most common cause of xerostomia. Over 500 prescription drugs list dry mouth as a potential side effect, and many OTC products cause dry mouth as well. Chronic disease such as Sjögren's syndrome or medical treatments for head and neck cancer commonly result in xerostomia as well. Left untreated, dry mouth can lead to increased dental caries, periodontal disease, dysphagia, and malnutrition. As a readily accessible HCP with expertise in both prescription and OTC medications, pharmacists are in a unique position to support patients suffering from dry mouth. Pharmacists can review medication histories to identify potential causes of dry mouth and offer guidance regarding symptomatic treatment and lifestyle modifications. Pharmacists can also identify and facilitate necessary referrals to other HCPs. An interdisciplinary approach to xerostomia is essential to ensure patients receive appropriate treatment for any underlying disease, potential modification of medications being used to treat comorbidities, and on-going management and support of xerostomia-related symptoms. Xerostomia is a common, yet often marginalized, patient complaint. An interdisciplinary approach to treatment offers the greatest opportunity for providing patients with symptomatic relief while preventing potential, serious complications.

REFERENCES

Abbasi, F., Farhadi, S., & Esmaili, M. (2013). Efficacy of pilocarpine and bromhexine in improving radiotherapy-induced xerostomia. *Journal of Dental Research, Dental Clinics, Dental Prospects, 7*(2), 86-90.

Alsakran Altamimi, M. A. (2014). Update knowledge of dry mouth—A guideline for dentists. *African Health Sciences, 14*(3), 736-742. doi:10.4314/ahs.v14i3.33

Araújo, J. R., & Martel, F. (2012). Sibutramine effects on central mechanisms regulating energy homeostasis. *Current Neuropharmacology, 10*(1), 49-52. doi:10.2174/157015912799362788

Centers for Disease Control and Prevention. (2018). Prescription drug use in the past 30 days, by sex, race and Hispanic origin, and age: United States, selected years 1988–1994 through 2011–2014. Retrieved from https://www.cdc.gov/nchs/hus/contents2017.htm#079

ClinCalc. (2018). Retrieved from https://clincalc.com/DrugStats/Top200Drugs.aspx

Clinical Pharmacology. (2018). Retrieved from http://www.clinicalpharmacology.com

Dagli, R. J., & Sharma, A. (2014). Polypharmacy: A global risk factor for elderly people. *Journal of International Oral Health, 6*(6), i-ii.

Delgado, A. J., & Olafsson, V. G. (2017). Acidic oral moisturizers with pH below 6.7 may be harmful to teeth depending on formulation: A short report. *Clinical, Cosmetic and Investigational Dentistry, 9*, 81-83. doi:10.2147/CCIDE.S140254

Donaldson, M., Epstein, J., & Villines, D. (2014). Managing the care of patients with Sjögren syndrome and dry mouth: Comorbidities, medication use and dental care considerations. *Journal of the American Dental Association, 145*(12), 1240-1247.

Erdemir, U., Okan, G., Gungor, S., Tekin, B., Yildiz, S. O., & Yildiz, E. (2017). The oral adverse effects of isotretinoin treatment in acne vulgaris patients: A prospective, case-control study. *Nigerian Journal of Clinical Practice, 20*(7), 860-866. doi:10.4103/1119-3077.183248

Femiano, F., Lanza, A., Buonaiuto, C., Gombos, F., Rullo, R., Festa, V., & Cirillo, N. (2008). Oral manifestations of adverse drug reactions: Guidelines. *Journal of the European Academy of Dermatology and Venereology, 22*(6), 681-691. doi:10.1111/j.1468-3083.2008.02637.x

Fife, R. S., Chase, W. F., Dore, R. K., Wiesenhutter, C. W., Lockhart, P. B., Tindall, E., & Suen, J. Y. (2002). Cevimeline for the treatment of xerostomia in patients with Sjögren syndrome: A randomized trial. *Archives of Internal Medicine, 162*(11), 1293-1300.

Fox, P. C. (2004). Salivary enhancement therapies. *Caries Research, 38*(3), 241-246. doi:10.1159/000077761

Frydrych, A. M. (2016). Dry mouth: Xerostomia and salivary gland hypofunction. *Australian Family Physician, 45*(7), 488-492.

Furness, S., Worthington, H. V., Bryan, G., Birchenough, S., McMillan, R. (2011). Interventions for the management of dry mouth: Topical therapies. *Cochrane Database of Systematic Reviews, 12*, CD008934. doi:10.1002/14651858.CD008934.pub2

Ghezzi, E. M., & Wagner-Lange, L. A. (2000). Longitudinal influence of age, menopause, hormone replacement therapy, and other medications on parotid flow rates in healthy women. *Journals of Gerontology Series A: Biological Sciences & Medical Sciences, 55*(1), M34-M42.

Goodrx.com. (n.d.a.). Pilocarpine. Retrieved from https://www.goodrx.com/pilocarpine?drug-name=pilocarpine

Goodrx.com. (n.d.b.). Cevimeline. Retrieved from https://www.goodrx.com/cevimeline

Götrick, B., & Tobin, G. (2004). The xerogenic potency and mechanism of action of tramadol inhibition of salivary secretion in rats. *Archives of Oral Biology, 49*(12), 969-973. doi:10.1016/j.archoralbio.2004.07.007

Gu, J., Zhu, S., Li, X., Wu, H., Li, Y., & Hua, F. (2014). Effect of amifostine in head and neck cancer patients treated with radiotherapy: A systematic review and meta-analysis based on randomized controlled trials. *PLOS One, 9*(5), e95968. doi:10.1371/journal.pone.0095968

Guggenheimer, J., & Moore, P. A. (2003). Xerostomia: Etiology, recognition and treatment. *Journal of the American Dental Association, 134*(1), 61-69.

Hahnel, S., Behr, M., Handel, G., & Bürgers, R. (2009). Saliva substitutes for the treatment of radiation-induced xerostomia—A review. *Supportive Care in Cancer, 17*(11), 1331-1343. doi:10.1007/s00520-009-0671-x

Hayes, C. (2001). The effect of non-cariogenic sweeteners on the prevention of dental caries: A review of the evidence. *Journal of Dental Education, 65*(10), 1106-1109.

Jensen, S. B., Pedersen, A. M., Vissink, A., Andersen, E., Brown, C. G., Davies, A. N., … Weikel, D. S. (2010). A systematic review of salivary gland hypofunction and xerostomia induced by cancer therapies: Prevalence, severity and impact on quality of life. *Supportive Care in Cancer, 18*(8), 1039-1060. doi:10.1007/s00520-010-0827-8

The Joint Commission. (2019). *National patient safety goals.* Retrieved from https://www.jointcommission.org/standards_information/npsgs.aspx

Kantor, E. D., Rehm, C. D., Haas, J. S., Chan, A. T., & Giovannucci, E. L. (2015). Trends in prescription drug use among adults in the United States from 1999-2012. *Journal of the American Medical Association, 314*(17), 1818-1831. doi:10.1001/jama.2015.13766

Kavitha, M., Mubeen, K., & Vijayalakshmi, K. R. (2017). A study on evaluation of efficacy of bethanechol in the management of chemoradiation-induced xerostomia in oral cancer patients. *Journal of Oral and Maxillofacial Pathology, 21*(3), 459-460.

Klotz, U. (2009). Pharmacokinetics and drug metabolism in the elderly. *Drug Metabolism Reviews, 41*(2), 67-76. doi:10.1080/03602530902722679

Kopach, O., Vats, J., Netsyk, O., Voitenko, N., Irving, A., & Fedirko, N. (2012). Cannabinoid receptors in submandibular acinar cells: Functional coupling between saliva fluid and electrolytes secretion and Ca2+ signaling. *Journal of Cell Science, 125*, 1884-1895. doi:10.1242/jcs.088930

Kubala, E., Strzelecka, P., Grzegocka, M., Lietz-Kijak, D., Gronwald, H., Skomro, P., & Kijak, E. (2018). A review of selected studies that determine the physical and chemical properties of saliva in the field of dental treatment. *BioMed Research International, 2018*, 1-13. doi:10.1155/2018/6572381

Lam, S., & Hilas, O. (2007). Pharmacologic management of overactive bladder. *Clinical Interventions in Aging, 2*(3), 337-345.

Lavan, A. H., & Gallagher, P. (2016). Predicting risk of adverse drug reactions in older adults. *Therapeutic Advances in Drug Safety, 7*(1), 11-22.

Lexicomp Online. (2018). Retrieved from http://online.lexi.com/lco/action/login

Mäkinen, K. K. (2016). Gastrointestinal disturbances associated with the consumption of sugar alcohols with special consideration of xylitol: Scientific review and instructions for dentists and other health-care professionals. *International Journal of Dentistry, 2016*, 5967907. doi:10.1155/2016/5967907

Millsop, J. W., Wang, E. A., & Fazel, N. (2017). Etiology, evaluation, and management of xerostomia. *Clinics in Dermatology, 35*(5), 468-476. doi:10.1016/j.clindermatol.2017.06.010

Miranda-Rius, J., Brunet-Llobet, L., Lahor-Soler, E., & Farré, M. (2015). Salivary secretory disorders, inducing drugs, and clinical management. *International Journal of Medical Sciences, 12*(10), 811-824. doi:10.7150/ijms.12912

Momm, F., Volegova-Neher, N. J., Schulte-Mönting, J., & Guttenberger, R. (2005). Different saliva substitutes for treatment of xerostomia following radiotherapy. A prospective crossover study. *Strahlentherapie Und Onkologie, 181*(4), 231-236.

Nadig, S. D., Ashwathappa, D. T., Manjunath, M., Krishna, S., Annaji, A. G., & Shivaprakash, P. K. (2017). A relationship between salivary flow rates and Candida counts in patients with xerostomia. *Journal of Oral and Maxillofacial Pathology, 21*(2), 316. doi:10.4103/jomfp.JOMFP_231_16

Napeñas, J. J., Brennan, M. T., & Fox, P. C. (2009). Diagnosis and treatment of xerostomia (dry mouth). *Odontology, 97*, 76-83. doi:10.1007/s10266-008-0099-7

Netherlands Pharmacovigilance Centre Lareb. (2013). Tamsulosin and dry mouth. Retrieved from https://databankws.lareb.nl/Downloads/KWB_2013_1_tamsu.pdf

Nieuw Amerongen, A. V., & Veerman, E. C. I. (2003). Current therapies for xerostomia and salivary gland hypofunction associated with cancer therapies. *Supportive Care in Cancer, 11*(4), 226-231.

Nguyen, C., MacEntee, M., Mintzes, B., & Perry, T. (2014). Information for physicians and pharmacists about drugs that might cause dry mouth: A study of monographs and published literature. *Drugs & Aging, 31*(1), 55-65. doi:10.1007/s40266-013-0141-5

Petrušić, N., Posavac, M., Sabol, I., & Mravak-Stipetić, M. (2015). The effect of tobacco smoking on salivation. *Acta Stomatologica Croatica, 49*(4), 309-315.

Plemons, J. M., Al-Hashimi, I., & Marek, C. L. (2014). Managing xerostomia and salivary gland hypofunction: Executive summary of a report from the American Dental Association Council on Scientific Affairs. *Journal of the American Dental Association, 145*(8), 867-873. doi: 10.14219/jada.2014.44

Porter, S. R., Scully, C., & Hegarty, A. M. (2004). An update of the etiology and management of xerostomia. *Oral Surgery, Oral Medicine, Oral Pathology, and Oral Radiology, 97*(1), 28-46. doi:j.tripleo.2003.07.010

Preetha, A., & Banerjee, R. (2005). Comparison of artificial saliva substitutes. *Trends in Biomaterials and Artificial Organs, 18*(2). Retrieved from http://medind.nic.in/taa/t05/i2/taat05i2p178.pdf

Proctor, G. B. (2016). The physiology of salivary secretion. *Periodontology 2000, 70*(1), 11-25. doi:10.1111/prd.12116

Rad, M., Kakoie, S., Niliye Brojeni, F., & Pourdamghan, N. (2010). Effect of long-term smoking on whole-mouth salivary flow rate and oral health. *Journal of Dental Research, Dental Clinics, Dental Prospects, 4*(4), 110-114.

Radvansky, L. J., Pace, M. B., & Siddiqui, A. (2013). Prevention and management of radiation-induced dermatitis, mucositis, and xerostomia. *American Journal of Health-System Pharmacy, 70*(12), 1025-1032. doi:10.2146/ajhp120467

Roganović, J. (2018). Pharmacodynamic causes of xerostomia in patients on psychotropic drugs. *ACTA Scientific Dental Sciences, 2*(11). Retrieved from https://actascientific.com/ASDS/pdf/ASDS-02-0350.pdf

Rommel, N., Rohleder, N. H., Koerdt, S., Wagenpfeil, S., Härtel-Petri, R., Wolff, K. D., & Kesting, M. R. (2016). Sympathomimetic effects of chronic methamphetamine abuse on oral health: A cross-sectional study. *BMC Oral Health, 16*(1), 59. doi:10.1186/s12903-016-0218-8

Sankar, V., & Rhodus, N. (2015). Dry mouth. The American Academy of Oral Medicine. Retrieved from https://www.aaom.com/dry-mouth

Scully, C. (2003). Drug effects on salivary glands: Dry mouth. *Oral Diseases, 9*(4), 165-176.

Scully, C., & Bagan, J. V. (2004). Adverse drug reactions in the orofacial region. *Critical Reviews in Oral Biology and Medicine, 15*(4), 221-239.

Scully, C., & Felix, D. H. (2005). Oral medicine—Update for the dental practitioner: Dry mouth and disorders of salivation. *British Dental Journal, 199*, 423-427.

Seitz, H. K., & Becker, P. (2007). Alcohol metabolism and cancer risk. *Alcohol Research & Health, 30*(1), 38-41, 44-47.

Sergi, G., De Rui, M., Sarti, S., & Manzato, E. (2011). Polypharmacy in the elderly: Can comprehensive geriatric assessment reduce inappropriate medication use? *Drugs & Aging, 28*(7), 509-518. doi:10.2165/11592010-000000000-00000

Ship, J. A. (2002). Diagnosis, managing, and preventing salivary gland disorders. *Oral Diseases, 8*(2), 77-89. doi:10.1034/j.1601-0825.2002.20837.x

Ship, J. A. (2003). Xerostomia in older adults: Diagnosis and management. *Oral Health, 6*(8), 44-48.

Smidt, D., Torpet, L. A., Nauntofte, B., Heegaard, K. M., & Pedersen, A. M. L. (2011). Associations between oral and ocular dryness, labial and whole salivary flow rates, systemic diseases and medications in a sample of older people. *Community Dentistry and Oral Epidemiology, 39*(3), 276-288. doi:10.1111/j.1600-0528.2010.00588.x

Sreebny, L. M., & Schwartz, S. S. (1997). A reference guide to drugs and dry mouth—2nd edition. *Gerontology, 14*(1), 33-47.

Tan, E. C. K., Lexomboon, D., Sandborgh-Englund, G., Haasum, Y., & Johnell, K. (2018). Medications that cause dry mouth as an adverse effect in older people: A systematic review and metaanalysis. *Journal of the American Geriatrics Society, 66*, 76-84. doi:10.1111/jgs.15151

Turner, M. D., & Ship, J. A. (2007). Dry mouth and its effects on the oral health of elderly people. *Journal of the American Dental Association, 138*(Suppl. 1), 15-20. doi:10.14219/jada.archive.2007.0358

United States Census Bureau. (2018). United States population projections 2000 to 2050. Retrieved from https://www.census.gov/library/working-papers/2009/demo/us-pop-proj-2000-2050.html

Villa, A., Connell, C., & Abati, S. (2015). Diagnosis and management of xerostomia and hyposalivation. *Therapeutics and Clinical Risk Management, 11*(1), 45-51. doi:10.2147/TCRM.S76282.

Wilcock, A., Twycross, R., Mortimer, J., & Thresiamma, M. P. (2006). Drug highlight: Pilocarpine. *Indian Journal of Palliative Care, 12*(2), 65-67. doi:10.4103/0973-1075.30247

Wiseman, L. R., & Faulds, D. (1995). Oral pilocarpine: A review of its pharmacological properties and clinical potential in xerostomia. *Drugs, 49*, 143. doi:10.2165/00003495-199549010-00010

Wolff, A., Joshi, R. K., Ekström, J., Aframian, D., Pedersen, A. M. L., Proctor, G., … Dawes, C. (2017). A guide to medications inducing salivary gland dysfunction, xerostomia, and subjective sialorrhea: A systematic review sponsored by the world workshop on oral medicine vi. *Drugs in R&D, 17*(1), 1-28. doi:10.1007/s40268-016-0153-9

World Health Organization Collaborating Centre for Drug Statistics Methodology. (2018). ATC classification index with DDDs. Retrieved from https://www.whocc.no/atc_ddd_index/

Wynn, R. L., & Meiller, T. F. (2001). Drugs and dry mouth. *General Dentistry, 49*(1), 10.

APPENDIX: DRUGS HAVING AN ADVERSE REACTION OF XEROSTOMIA

- Abciximab
- Abemaciclib
- AbobotulinumtoxinA
- Acetaminophen/butalbital
- Acetaminophen/butalbital/caffeine
- Acetaminophen/butalbital/caffeine/codeine
- Acetaminophen/caffeine/dihydrocodeine
- Acetaminophen/caffeine/magnesium salicylate/phenyltoloxamine
- Acetaminophen/caffeine/phenyltoloxamine/salicylamide
- Acetaminophen/chlorpheniramine/dextromethorphan/phenylephrine
- Acetaminophen/chlorpheniramine/dextromethorphan/pseudoephedrine
- Acetaminophen/chlorpheniramine/phenylephrine/phenyltoloxamine
- Acetaminophen/dextromethorphan/doxylamine
- Acetaminophen/dextromethorphan/guaifenesin/phenylephrine
- Acetaminophen/dextromethorphan/phenylephrine
- Acetaminophen/dextromethorphan/pseudoephedrine
- Acetaminophen/diphenhydramine
- Acetaminophen/hydrocodone
- Acetaminophen/oxycodone
- Acetaminophen/tramadol
- Acetazolamide
- Acitretin
- Aclidinium
- Acrivastine/pseudoephedrine
- Adenosine
- Ado-trastuzumab emtansine
- Agalsidase beta
- Albuterol
- Albuterol/ipratropium
- Aliskiren/amlodipine
- Aliskiren/amlodipine/hydrochlorothiazide
- Almotriptan
- Alosetron
- Alprazolam
- Alprostadil
- Amantadine
- Amikacin
- Amiloride
- Amiloride/hydrochlorothiazide
- Amitriptyline

- Amitriptyline/chlordiazepoxide
- Amlodipine
- Amlodipine/benazepril
- Amlodipine/celecoxib
- Amlodipine/hydrochlorothiazide/valsartan
- Amlodipine/valsartan
- Amoxapine
- Amoxicillin/clarithromycin/omeprazole
- Amoxicillin/clarithromycin/lansoprazole
- Amphetamine
- Amphetamine/dextroamphetamine
- Amphotericin B cholesteryl sulfate complex
- Amphotericin B liposomal
- Anastrozole
- Apraclonidine
- Aprepitant/fosaprepitant
- Arformoterol
- Aripiprazole
- Armodafinil
- Arsenic trioxide
- Articaine/epinephrine
- Asenapine
- Aspirin/butalbital/caffeine/codeine
- Aspirin/omeprazole
- Aspirin/oxycodone
- Astemizole
- Atenolol
- Atenolol/chlorthalidone
- Atomoxetine
- Atropine
- Atropine/benzoic acid/hyoscyamine/methenamine/methylene blue/phenyl salicylate
- Atropine/difenoxin
- Atropine/diphenoxylate
- Atropine/edrophonium
- Atropine/hyoscyamine/phenobarbital/scopolamine
- Axicabtagene ciloleucel
- Azelastine
- Azelastine/fluticasone
- Baclofen
- Balsalazide
- Beclomethasone
- Belladonna alkaloids/ergotamine/phenobarbital
- Belladonna/opium
- Benazepril/hydrochlorothiazide

- Bendamustine
- Bendroflumethiazide/nadolol
- Benznidazole
- Benzoic acid/hyoscyamine/methenamine/methylene blue/phenyl salicylate
- Benzphetamine
- Benztropine
- Bepridil
- Betaxolol
- Bexarotene
- Bicalutamide
- Bismuth subcitrate potassium/metronidazole/tetracycline
- Bismuth subsalicylate/metronidazole/tetracycline
- Bisoprolol
- Bisoprolol/hydrochlorothiazide
- Boceprevir
- Brexpiprazole
- Brimonidine
- Brimonidine/brinzolamide
- Brimonidine/timolol
- Brinzolamide
- Bromocriptine
- Brompheniramine
- Brompheniramine/carbetapentane/phenylephrine
- Brompheniramine/dextromethorphan/guaifenesin
- Brompheniramine/guaifenesin/hydrocodone
- Brompheniramine/hydrocodone/pseudoephedrine
- Brompheniramine/pseudoephedrine
- Budesonide
- Bumetanide
- Buprenorphine
- Bupropion
- Bupropion/naltrexone
- Busulfan
- Butorphanol
- Cabergoline
- Calcifediol
- Calcitonin
- Calcitriol
- Calcium/vitamin D
- Canagliflozin
- Canagliflozin/metformin
- Capecitabine
- Captopril
- Captopril/hydrochlorothiazide

- Carbamazepine
- Carbenicillin
- Carbetapentane/chlorpheniramine
- Carbetapentane/chlorpheniramine/phenylephrine
- Carbetapentane/diphenhydramine/phenylephrine
- Carbetapentane/phenylephrine/pyrilamine
- Carbetapentane/pyrilamine
- Carbidopa/levodopa
- Carbidopa/levodopa/entacapone
- Carbinoxamine
- Carbinoxamine/dextromethorphan/pseudoephedrine
- Carbinoxamine/hydrocodone/phenylephrine
- Carbinoxamine/hydrocodone/pseudoephedrine
- Carbinoxamine/phenylephrine
- Carbinoxamine/pseudoephedrine
- Carboprost tromethamine
- Cariprazine
- Carisoprodol
- Carvedilol
- Cefdinir
- Cefditoren
- Cefpodoxime
- Ceftibuten
- Celecoxib
- Cephalothin
- Cetirizine
- Cetirizine/pseudoephedrine
- Cetuximab
- Cevimeline
- Chlophedianol/dexchlorpheniramine/pseudoephedrine
- Chlorcyclizine
- Chlordiazepoxide/clidinium
- Chlorhexidine
- Chlorpheniramine
- Chlorpheniramine/codeine
- Chlorpheniramine/dextromethorphan
- Chlorpheniramine/dextromethorphan/phenylephrine
- Chlorpheniramine/dihydrocodeine/phenylephrine
- Chlorpheniramine/dihydrocodeine/pseudoephedrine
- Chlorpheniramine/guaifenesin/hydrocodone/pseudoephedrine
- Chlorpheniramine/hydrocodone
- Chlorpheniramine/hydrocodone/phenylephrine

- Chlorpheniramine/hydrocodone/pseudoephedrine
- Chlorpheniramine/phenylephrine
- Chlorpheniramine/pseudoephedrine
- Chlorpromazine
- Chlorthalidone/clonidine
- Ciclesonide
- Cidofovir
- Ciprofloxacin
- Citalopram
- Clarithromycin
- Clemastine
- Clomipramine
- Clonidine
- Clorazepate
- Clozapine
- Cod liver oil
- Codeine
- Codeine/phenylephrine/promethazine
- Codeine/promethazine
- Creatine
- Crofelemer
- Cyclizine
- Cyclobenzaprine
- Cyclopentolate
- Cyclosporine
- Cyproheptadine
- Daptomycin
- Darifenacin
- Daunorubicin liposomal
- Delavirdine
- Desipramine
- Desloratadine
- Desloratadine/pseudoephedrine
- Desmopressin
- Desvenlafaxine
- Deutetrabenazine
- Dexchlorpheniramine
- Dexchlorpheniramine/dextromethorphan/pseudoephedrine
- Dexfenfluramine
- Dexlansoprazole
- Dexmedetomidine
- Dexmethylphenidate
- Dextroamphetamine

- Dextromethorphan/diphenhydramine/phenylephrine
- Dextromethorphan/promethazine
- Diazepam
- Diazoxide
- Diclofenac
- Diclofenac/misoprostol
- Dicyclomine
- Didanosine
- Diethylpropion
- Dihydrocodeine/guaifenesin/pseudoephedrine
- Dihydroergotamine
- Diltiazem
- Dimenhydrinate
- Diphenhydramine
- Diphenhydramine/hydrocodone/phenylephrine
- Diphenhydramine/ibuprofen
- Diphenhydramine/phenylephrine
- Dipyridamole
- Disopyramide
- Dorzolamide
- Dorzolamide/timolol
- Doxazosin
- Doxepin
- Doxercalciferol
- Doxycycline
- Doxylamine
- Doxylamine/pyridoxine
- Duloxetine
- Dutasteride/tamsulosin
- Echinacea
- Eletriptan
- Enalapril
- Enalapril/hydrochlorothiazide
- Enfuvirtide
- Entacapone
- Ephedra
- Eprosartan
- Ertapenem
- Escitalopram
- Esmolol
- Esomeprazole
- Estazolam
- Eszopiclone
- Etodolac

- Etravirine
- Everolimus
- Ezogabine
- Famotidine
- Febuxostat
- Felbamate
- Fenfluramine
- Fenofibrate
- Fenoprofen
- Fentanyl
- Fesoterodine
- Fexofenadine/pseudoephedrine
- Flavoxate
- Flecainide
- Flibanserin
- Fluconazole
- Flucytosine
- Flumazenil
- Flunisolide
- Fluocinolone/hydroquinone/tretinoin
- Fluoxetine
- Fluoxetine/olanzapine
- Fluphenazine
- Flurazepam
- Flurbiprofen
- Fluticasone
- Fluticasone/salmeterol
- Fluticasone/umeclidinium/vilanterol
- Fluvoxamine
- Formoterol
- Foscarnet
- Fosfomycin
- Fosinopril
- Fosinopril/hydrochlorothiazide
- Fosphenytoin
- Frovatriptan
- Gabapentin
- Gadobenate/dimeglumine
- Gadobutrol
- Gadopentetate
- Gadoteridol
- Gadoversetamide
- Gadoxetate disodium
- Ganciclovir

- Gefitinib
- Gemifloxacin
- Glatiramer
- Glycopyrrolate
- Glycopyrrolate/formoterol
- Glycopyrronium
- Goserelin
- Grepafloxacin
- Guaifenesin/hydrocodone
- Guaifenesin/hydrocodone/pseudoephedrine
- Guaifenesin/phenylephrine
- Guanabenz
- Guanfacine
- Guanidine
- Haloperidol
- Homatropine hydrobromide
- Homatropine/hydrocodone
- Hydrochlorothiazide/lisinopril
- Hydrochlorothiazide/losartan
- Hydrochlorothiazide/methyldopa
- Hydrochlorothiazide/metoprolol
- Hydrochlorothiazide/moexipril
- Hydrochlorothiazide/triamterene
- Hydrochlorothiazide/valsartan
- Hydrocodone
- Hydrocodone/ibuprofen
- Hydrocodone/potassium guaiacolsulfonate
- Hydrocodone/potassium guaiacolsulfonate/pseudoephedrine
- Hydromorphone
- Hydroxyzine
- Hyoscyamine
- Hyoscyamine/methenamine/methylene blue/phenyl salicylate/sodium biphosphate
- Ibuprofen
- Ibuprofen/oxycodone
- Iloperidone
- Imatinib
- Imipramine
- IncobotulinumtoxinA
- Indacaterol
- Indapamide
- Inotersen
- Interferon alfa-2B
- Interferon alfa-2B/ribavirin
- Interferon alfa-n3

- Interferon beta-1a
- Iobenguane I 131
- Iodixanol
- Iohexol
- Iopamidol
- Iopromide
- Ioversol
- Ipratropium
- Isocarboxazid
- Isosorbide dinitrate
- Isosorbide mononitrate
- Isotretinoin
- Ketoprofen
- Ketorolac
- Lacosamide
- Lamotrigine
- Lansoprazole
- Lansoprazole/naproxen
- Leflunomide
- Lenalidomide
- Lenvatinib
- Letrozole
- Leuprolide
- Levalbuterol
- Levocabastine
- Levocetirizine
- Levomethadyl
- Levorphanol
- L-glutamine
- Liraglutide
- Lisdexamfetamine
- Lisinopril
- Lithium
- Lofexidine
- Lomefloxacin
- Loperamide
- Loperamide/simethicone
- Lopinavir/ritonavir
- Loratadine
- Loratadine/pseudoephedrine
- Lorcaserin
- Losartan
- Lovastatin
- Loxapine

- Lurasidone
- Mannitol
- Mannitol/sorbitol
- Maprotiline
- Marijuana/medical
- Meclizine
- Mefenamic acid
- Megestrol
- Meloxicam
- Mepenzolate
- Meperidine
- Meperidine/promethazine
- Mesna
- Mesoridazine
- Metaproterenol
- Methadone
- Methamphetamine
- Methazolamide
- Methenamine/sodium acid phosphate/methylene blue/hyoscyamine
- Methscopolamine
- Methyldopa
- Methylene blue
- Methylphenidate
- Metolazone
- Metoprolol
- Metronidazole
- Metyrosine
- Mexiletine
- Miconazole
- Midodrine
- Mifepristone
- Miglustat
- Milnacipran
- Minocycline
- Mirabegron
- Mirtazapine
- Mixed grass pollens allergen extract
- Modafinil
- Moexipril
- Molindone
- Mometasone
- Morphine
- Morphine/naltrexone
- Moxifloxacin

- Mupirocin
- Mycophenolate
- Nabilone
- Nabumetone
- Nadolol
- Nalbuphine
- Naltrexone
- Naproxen
- Naproxen/sumatriptan
- Nefazodone
- Neostigmine
- Neratinib
- Netupitant/fosnetupitant/palonosetron
- Nicardipine
- Nicotine
- Nifedipine
- Nilotinib
- Nilutamide
- Niraparib
- Nitazoxanide
- Nitroglycerin
- Nizatidine
- Norfloxacin
- Nortriptyline
- Obiltoxaximab
- Ofloxacin
- Olanzapine
- Olopatadine
- Olsalazine
- Omacetaxine
- Omeprazole
- Omeprazole/sodium bicarbonate
- OnabotulinumtoxinA
- Orphenadrine
- Oxaliplatin
- Oxaprozin
- Oxcarbazepine
- Oxybutynin
- Oxycodone
- Oxycodone/naloxone
- Oxycodone/naltrexone
- Oxymorphone
- Paliperidone
- Palonosetron

- Panitumumab
- Panobinostat
- Pantoprazole
- Paricalcitol
- Paroxetine
- Peginterferon alfa-2a
- Peginterferon alfa-2b
- Pentamidine
- Pentazocine
- Pentazocine/naloxone
- Pentoxifylline
- Perflutren lipid microspheres
- Perflutren protein-type A microspheres
- Pergolide
- Perindopril/amlodipine
- Perphenazine
- Perphenazine/amitriptyline
- Phendimetrazine
- Phenelzine
- Phentermine
- Phentermine/topiramate
- Phenylephrine/promethazine
- Phenylpropanolamine
- Phenytoin
- Pilocarpine
- Pimozide
- Pirbuterol
- Piroxicam
- Plerixafor
- Pralidoxime
- Pramipexole
- Prazosin
- Pregabalin
- Procarbazine
- Prochlorperazine
- Promethazine
- Propafenone
- Propantheline
- Propofol
- Protriptyline
- Quazepam
- Quetiapine
- Quinapril
- Rabeprazole

- Ramipril
- Ranolazine
- Rasagiline
- Reboxetine
- Remifentanil
- Reserpine
- Ribavirin
- Ribociclib
- Rifapentine
- Riluzole
- RimabotulinumtoxinB
- Rimantadine
- Risperidone
- Rizatriptan
- Rofecoxib
- Ropinirole
- Rotigotine
- S-adenosyl-L-methionine
- Salmeterol
- Saquinavir
- Scopolamine
- Selegiline
- Sertraline
- Sevoflurane
- Short ragweed pollen allergen extract
- Sibutramine
- Sildenafil
- Simethicone
- Sodium ferric gluconate complex/ferric pyrophosphate citrate
- Sodium iodide I 131
- Sodium oxybate
- Solifenacin
- Sorafenib
- Sorbitol
- Sparfloxacin
- St. John's wort (*Hypericum perforatum*)
- Sucralfate
- Sugammadex
- Sulindac
- Sumatriptan
- Sunitinib
- Suvorexant
- Tacrine
- Tacrolimus

- Tadalafil
- Tamsulosin
- Tapentadol
- Tecovirimat
- Telithromycin
- Terazosin
- Terbutaline
- Terfenadine
- Testosterone
- Thalidomide
- Thiabendazole
- Thiethylperazine
- Thioridazine
- Thithixene
- Tiagabine
- Tiludronate
- Timothy grass pollen allergen extract
- Tinidazole
- Tiotropium
- Tiotropium/olodaterol
- Tizanidine
- Tolcapone
- Tolterodine
- Tolvaptan
- Topiramate
- Torsemide
- Tramadol
- Trametinib
- Trandolapril
- Trandolapril/verapamil
- Tranylcypromine
- Trazodone
- Triamcinolone
- Triamterene
- Triazolam
- Trifluoperazine
- Trihexyphenidyl
- Trimipramine
- Triprolidine
- Tropicamide
- Trospium
- Umeclidinium
- Umeclidinium/vilanterol
- Unoprostone

- Valbenazine
- Valproic acid/divalproex sodium
- Valsartan
- Vandetanib
- Vardenafil
- Varenicline
- Venlafaxine
- Verapamil
- Vilazodone
- Voriconazole
- Vortioxetine
- Zaleplon
- Ziconotide
- Ziprasidone
- Zoledronic acid
- Zolmitriptan
- Zolpidem
- Zonisamide

Adapted from ClinCalc (2018), Clinical Pharmacology (2018), and Lexicomp Online, (2018).

FINANCIAL DISCLOSURES

Dr. Rebecca H. Affoo has no financial or proprietary interest in the materials presented herein.

Dr. Michael A. Blasco has no financial or proprietary interest in the materials presented herein.

Dr. Yusuf Dundar has no financial or proprietary interest in the materials presented herein.

Dr. Lea E. Erickson has no financial or proprietary interest in the materials presented herein.

Dr. Sarah M. Ginsberg has no financial or proprietary interest in the materials presented herein.

Dr. Jeffrey M. Hotaling has no financial or proprietary interest in the materials presented herein.

Dr. Sharon Ingersoll has no financial or proprietary interest in the materials presented herein.

Dr. Joseph Murray has no financial or proprietary interest in the materials presented herein.

Dr. Kristine Tanner has no financial or proprietary interest in the materials presented herein.

Dr. Bryan Trump has no financial or proprietary interest in the materials presented herein.

INDEX

Printed in the United States
by Baker & Taylor Publisher Services